STRESS IN INDUSTRY

Accidents at work cause an average loss of 23 million working days in a year—but days lost through various forms of mental stress and resulting illnesses exceed 37 million. Mental illness is now the second fastest growing cause of absence from work. An international seminar on industrial stress was arranged at Windsor Castle two years ago on behalf of the World Federation for Mental Health. One of the organisers was Dr. Joseph Kearns and his book is a direct result of that exercise in prevention.

In his Foreword, the Rt. Hon. David Ennals—a former Minister of State for Health and Social Security and now Director of the MIND Campaign of the National Association for Mental Health—says "This is quite the best diagnosis of stress factors at work that I have read . . . I commend it to management, trades unions and all who have responsibility for people at work".

Dr. Kearns analyses many aspects of work stress, from the manager's career—building worries to group stress on the factory floor. By bringing together the knowledge gained so far, not only in this country but also in the United States and a number of European countries, Dr. Kearns succeeds in showing how industrial stress can be tackled at organisation, trades union and national levels. His book will also help doctors to recognise and treat stress illnesses.

Joseph Kearns was educated at St. Benedict's Abbey, Ealing, and is a graduate of University College, Dublin. Joe Kearns enjoyed the usual sequence of experience in hospital and National Service Medicine to succeed his father in general practice in Shepherds Bush, London. After several years as a principal in a rapidly developing practice, he took the opportunity to enter Ocupational Medicine.

Active in medical politics and a member of the British Medical Association, Dr. Kearns has also contributed to activities both of the Royal College of General Practitioners and the Society of Occupational Medicine.

PRIORY EDITORIAL CONSULTANTS

THE CARE AND WELFARE LIBRARY

Consultant Medical Editor A. R. K. Mitchell,
MB, Ch.B, MRCPE, MRCPsych.

STRESS IN INDUSTRY

JOSEPH L. KEARNS
MB, BCh., MSc.

Group Medical Adviser, J. Lyons Group of Companies

Foreword by

The Rt Hon DAVID ENNALS

Director of the MIND Campaign of the National
Association for Mental Health and formerly Minister
of State for Health and Social Security

PRIORY PRESS LIMITED

The Care and Welfare Library

SBN 85078 054 3 (Hardback)
       85078 055 1 (Paperback)
Copyright © 1973 by Joseph Kearns
First published in 1973 by
Priory Press Limited
101 Grays Inn Road London WC1
Made and printed in Great Britain by
The Garden City Press Limited
Letchworth, Hertfordshire SG6 1JS

Acknowledgements

MY thanks are due to Mr. David Ennals for his Foreword to the book, and to Dr. Roger Tredgold and Dr. J. Aldridge, the other two organisers of the seminar referred to in the Preface. Together with me they edited the Proceedings of that seminar, and they encouraged me to undertake this task. Illustrations of Hector the Hedgehog are based upon drawings by Mrs. I. Campbell, SRN.

The Gulf Publishing Company, the University of Minnesota, the Industrial Society, and PULSE gave permission for use of the Grid Diagram, the paper on T-groups, the illustration of Maslow's Hierarchy, and the cartoon on page 157. The review of literature in the chapter on Absenteeism is taken from the author's unpublished MSC. project.

Acknowledgement is due to Interpharma, whose initial grant made the Windsor seminar possible. My thanks are also due to Mrs. D. McKie, my secretary, who typed and retyped the text—not without complaint, but always with good humour.

Finally, the International Committee on Occupational Mental Health is grateful to Dr. Geoffrey Eley, Editorial Director of Priory Press Ltd. Had he not discovered—and appreciated—the original seminar proceedings this book would not have appeared.

Contents

Foreword

The Rt. Hon. David Ennals, Director of the MIND Campaign of the National Association for Mental Health.

THIS book by Dr. Joseph Kearns comes at a very appropriate time. In 1970 Lord Robens and a small committee were asked by the Secretary of State for Employment to study the whole question of 'Safety and Health at Work'. Their report was published in July 1972 and to the disappointment of many people, it totally ignored psychological factors in the work situation.

The report seemed to be concerned only with physical health and safety and based its studies on the fact that on average there were 23,000,000 working days lost through accidents at work— ignoring the fact that, in 1969/70, days lost from psychosis, psycho-neurosis, nervousness, debility and headaches totalled nearly 37,000,000. Even these figures, based on sickness absence notes, underestimates the size of the problems of stress factors affecting work performance, for it excludes dyspepsia, skin com- plaints and muscular aches and pains which are increasingly recognised as symptoms of stress. As the Office of Health Economics recently pointed out 'it is increasingly recognised that conditions like "bronchitis" or "slipped disc" are simply used as conventional diagnostic labels for episodes of absence which often owe more to social and economic factors than a simple inability to work for medical reasons. Rising (sickness) absence rates probably reflect, above all else, a lack of satisfaction at work. . . ."

The Robens Report ignores also the steady growth in voluntary absenteeism, not covered by sickness notes, which illustrates an increase in job dissatisfaction and a decrease in identification with

the job in hand. Rising absence rates—from whatever cause—
certainly do not reflect an increase in the amount of sickness in
the community as a whole. In 1970 certified sickness absence
accounted for 342,000,000 days—an increase of nine million on
1969 and a rise of 22 per cent in the past fifteen years. In the same
period, days lost through psycho-neurosis and psychosis increased
by 152 per cent for men and 302 per cent for women. Looked at
over this fifteen-year time span, mental illness is now the second
fastest growing cause of days lost from work. It claims more working days than 'flu and the common cold together and more than
the whole range of accidents. In 1970 it accounted for more than
three times the amount of time lost through industrial disputes.

This book by Dr. Kearns puts the whole subject of stress at
work into perspective—and valuably draws on experience in
other countries—especially the campaign which was launched in
Sweden in 1968 to involve workers and management in a study
of the effects of internal and external factors on mental health
within working life.

The seminar at Windsor in 1970, on which this book is based,
owes something to the initiative of the National Association for
Mental Health and what I find fascinating is that, though the
team of experts who pooled their knowledge at the seminar are
in almost every case different from those who came together at
my invitation to prepare our evidence to the Robens Committee,
their conclusions, as reflected in Dr. Kearns' book, are the same.

In our evidence we highlighted five danger points. Firstly,
overpromotion : stress, anxiety and often breakdown can follow
from responsibilities beyond a person's capacities. Secondly,
underwork : sometimes agreeable for a time but leads to dissatisfaction, doubts about the worker's capacities, demoralisation
and frequent spells of absence for minor complaints. Thirdly,
job definition : it is essential that the employee should know the
requirements of the job and to whom he is responsible. Uncertainty over these issues can become a major strain. The resulting
stress can be taken by seniors as implying inadequacy for the job,
when the real cause of trouble is lack of clarity by higher
management.

The fourth danger point is lack of effective *consultation and communication*—an all too common fault of management. Sudden unexplained changes in policy, take-overs and fears of redundancy can cause stress disorders. There is a correlation between the level of morale of employees and the quality of concern of senior management for the people they employ. And, fifth on our list, we pointed out that many manual workers have no *financial security* from their employers such as job security, sick pay or pension schemes, which the clerical and management groups largely take for granted. This has obvious deleterious effects upon the psychological and physical health of these workers.

The need for the establishment of an Occupational Health Service was also emphasised in N.A.M.H.'s evidence to Robens. We proposed that it should be a statutory service, linked with the N.H.S., providing for all the working population not covered by existing industrial health schemes. The occupational health teams should consist of physicians, nurses, welfare officers and social workers and should work closely with the G.P. service. Such a team could help in the early identification of stress symptoms and would be better able than a G.P. alone to relate the individual's state of health to the job he has to perform. Moreover, they would be able to advise management on ways of minimising unnecessary stress and conflict.

This proposal goes further than Dr. Kearns—but this book is quite the best diagnosis of stress factors at work that I have read. I commend it to Lord Robens and his committee—as well as to management, trades unions and all who have responsibility for people at work.

Preface

THIS book has two objectives; to respond to the demand for more copies of the Proceedings of a Seminar on "Stress in Industry", and to satisfy one of the declared aims of that seminar in providing information to the wider non-technical audience who may be victims of stress, and may perhaps even cause it.

The volume of literature on the subject is already vast. A great deal of it is technical and is directed to social scientists, psychologists, behavioural scientists and a host of others whose specialism is directed to improving the lot of those considered to be under-privileged or under-educated, and of individuals under-valued by the society in which they live. This book is a modest attempt to explain in broad terms, to the community at large, the stresses we provoke in others; the effects that other individuals and organisations may have on each of us; and the practical steps that might be taken to reduce the harm done to others. Each chapter can be read on its own, or in relation to other chapters in the book. The list of references is intended to signpost further information for the reader with an interest in a particular aspect of stress.

In 1964 a number of people in different professions, coming mainly from North West Europe, set up the International Committee on Occupational Mental Health. The discipline of a meeting for a few days each year gives this group a stimulus to consider some topic, which becomes the theme of discussions. In 1969 Interpharma, a consortium of pharmaceutical companies based in Switzerland, sponsored the study of mental health by the World Federation for Mental Health. Through the agency of the National Association for Mental Health in the United Kingdom, the World Federation asked the British members of the

International Committee on Occupational Mental Health to organise a seminar on Stress in Industry, which took place in St. George's House, Windsor Castle in the summer of 1970.

That particular seminar was designed to have some product, and the Proceedings have been well received. What was originally considered to be a very ambitious edition of 500 copies has been sold out to individuals and organisations in many parts of the world, and demand continues. Events since the seminar took place afford an opportunity to re-edit and expand the original material on a greater scale than any of the organisers would have originally expected. I am grateful to the ten authors who led discussion in the seminar on the topics listed in this Preface. They have generously consented to my plagiarising their work. The other participants have not been individually approached, but the spirit of their contribution and the intentions and hopes expressed at the end of the seminar, lead me to believe that they will have no objection to my attempt to convey the results of their work to a wider audience. The "workshop" structure of the seminar produced "group" results of which the story of Hector the Hedgehog is but one example.

In the scientific sense, there is little in the book for which I can claim original credit. I have already attempted to set this book in the context of other written work. Let me persuade those interested in this subject that "cognitive" learning derived from books is insufficient without the experience of informed observations of interpersonal and intergroup behaviour as it takes place. Such "experiential" courses in human behaviour are few in relation to the need for them, because trainers are both scarce and expensive and tend to focus attention on problems which attract managers, rather than those managed. The chapter describing courses directed to the whole working population of Sweden may suggest to us how we in the U.K. might overcome the shortage of trainers, organise study groups at a less sophisticated level than those now available, and direct the attention of "ordinary" people to some of the problems that confront them.

I make no apology for repeating what has been said before, to specialist audiences. I merely hope to tell the reader what other people know about him, and what he should know about himself.

THE WINDSOR SEMINAR 1970

Discussion Leaders	Subject
R. Markillie, Consultant Psychiatrist, University of Leeds, England	Organisational factors causing stress
R. F. Tredgold, Consultant Psychiatrist, University College Hospital, London	Stress reactions in the individual
T. G. P. Rogers, Director of External Affairs, I.B.M. (United Kingdom) Limited	The Manager's stress
J. Bannister, Senior Shop Steward, Transport and General Workers' Union	Stress on the shop floor
E. Mindus, Chief Medical Officer, Statens Vagverk, Sweden	A national mental health campaign
J. Doeglas, Psychologist, Philips Gloeilampenfabrieken	A company's mental health campaign
R. Murray, Medical Adviser, Trades Union Congress, London	Union attitudes to mental health
O. Maček, Professor, Dept. of Occupational Medicine, Sarajevo, Yugoslavia	Problems of education in mental health
A. Brook, Consultant Psychiatrist, Cassel Hospital, Richmond, England	Training British doctors in industrial mental health
B. Neale, Personnel Manager, I.C.I., London	An approach to management

Other participants, and their roles at the time
of the seminar

J. Aldridge, Medical Adviser, IB.M. (United Kingdom) Ltd.
M. Braaten, Medical Officer, Kongsberg Vapenfabrikk, Norway
H. Bridger, Programme Director, Dept. of Career Development,
Tavistock Institute of Human Relations, London

R. Brough, Psychologist, Port of New York Authority, U.S.A.

T. Carruthers, Psychologist, University of Glasgow

G. di Elia, Psychologist, S.A. Uff. Formazione e Documentazione, Milan

C. Doyle, Medical Correspondent, *The Observer*, London

A. Hirschfield, Lecturer, University of Michigan, U.S.A.

R. Hirschfield, Consultant Psychiatrist, Michigan, U.S.A.

H. Holden, Medical Officer, British Insulated Callender's Cables, England

J. Kearns, Medical Adviser, J. Lyons Group of Companies, England

A. de Kretser, Medical Officer, Vauxhall Motors, Luton, England

J. Kuiper, Medical Adviser to Ministry of Social Affairs, Breda, Holland

A. Muirhead, Medical Adviser, British Broadcasting Corporation

G. Nerell, Medical Officer, L.M. Ericsam, Stockholm, Sweden

F. Novara, Lecturer in Occupational Psychology, University of Turin, Italy

K. Osborne, Industrial Relations Adviser, J. Lyons Group of Companies, England

H. Rhee, Sociologist, Geneva

A. Roberts, Management Consultant, London

C. Smith, Consultant Physician, Dublin

G. Ter Veroorde, Psychologist, Philips Gloeilampenfabrieken, Eindhoven, Holland

P. Verhaegen, Professor of Psychology, Katholieke, Universiteit te Leuven, Belgium

A. Weir, Lecturer in Psychology, University of Glasgow

Information about the International Committee on Occupational Mental Health is available from the Secretary: Dr. J. D. A. Doeglas, Philips Gloeilampenfabrieken, Eindhoven, Netherlands.

I

Prevention

THE Windsor seminar, upon which most of the material in this book is based, was called "an exercise in prevention" a phrase which has two interpretations.

The organisers had set out to draw together people in different professions, from different cultural backgrounds, in the hope that their efforts would suggest a practical programme for the prevention—or at least diminution—of stress in industrial organisations. Rather than meet to hear papers read, material intended to lead discussion was circulated before the meeting, and members were then expected to work in four small groups, each group being a mixture of representatives of nations and professions. This "workshop" design justified another interpretation of the subtitle "an exercise in prevention", because individuals who had not worked together before experienced stress themselves.

Any meeting between people is made up of content and process. The content is made up of the debate itself, the arguments for and against, the facts and figures, and all the material which might be mentioned in an agenda. The process of a meeting, which in some senses is an agenda which is not apparent though none the less real, is that activity represented by attempts to establish or dispute leadership of the meeting, the awareness by the debater and others of his status, the scoring of points in argument, and all those events not confined to the merits of the subject under discussion, but forming the political manoeuvring between those debating it.

The different disciplines represented noted that stress was assumed to occur predominantly in managerial and technical staff, and there was some conflict generated by the assertion that manual workers and skilled craftsmen also suffered. At times, within the groups, those who could be described as "technical" seemed almost to dispute the possibility that those further down the Registrar General's grades of social class possessed sufficient intellectual sophistication to be aware of stress. The reverse was also true, in that representatives of trades unions appeared at times to lay claim to a "right" to be stressed as much as others who had had the advantage of higher education. Neither side disputed that stress could be experienced by anybody, but both sides seemed at times to be discussing the status bestowed by being subjected to stressors.

This conflict between groups representing technical and skilled people was complicated by conflicts between different though sometimes overlapping groupings. Some participants had known each other for years before the meeting, others were strangers meeting for the first time. Single strangers evidently felt threatened by the presence of acquainted groups; that is to say that a newcomer who considered himself to be an expert, and whose expertise had been recognised in his own community, feared that views he would express might be opposed by a pre-existing group of perhaps only two old friends, who enjoyed the advantage of each other's recognition, while the stranger could only hope for support from other strangers in the group. Anxiety in expressing expertise was thus magnified by fear of numbers for and against, of "losing", and being seen to lose.

Paradoxically this anxiety sometimes led to a speaker taking refuge in indefiniteness because an indefinite statement is less open to challenge than one that is definite. A further complication was the use of colloquial English, so that a third overlapping grouping reflected those familiar with English, and others who were themselves further divided by their own native tongues. Emotion, insistence on status, denial by others of that claimed status, and hesitation before attempting to express an opinion in a foreign tongue were all early obstacles to be overcome.

As relations improved, and as attention was increasingly being focused upon the content of the debate, each of the groups became aware of problems of communication. It will be no surprise to read that between countries, the same word could have very different meanings. The term "manager" in Britain would describe anyone who had a number of people in his charge, but in Holland the word would imply a very senior post in an organisation. Differences of organisation also became apparent, and these confusing terms and philosophies were found to exist even within one nation.

As the discussion process continued, certain types of behaviour were seen to have significant effects upon the ease of communication. One of these was the personal establishment of one's own status by claiming a particular expertise. A person referred to his own original work and experience, claimed superior knowledge, or monopolised conversation with anecdote after anecdote. This behaviour was accompanied by disarming phrases such as "of course, everyone is familiar with . . .", or "I don't want to talk too much", or again "our country hasn't anything special to teach . . .". Such insincere and even untrue statements only increased resistance to the individual concerned by the rest of his group, with a resulting increase in tension. In one group, paralysis of communication was so complete that an infuriated foreigner, normally a fluent English speaker, found himself utterly unable to express himself at all.

Subsequently, all members of the group were encouraged to express their personal frustrations, so that greater understanding and sympathy were both felt and expressed. The more friendly atmosphere made it less necessary for any member of the group to be so defensive, or even aggressive, and debate flowed more freely. Three areas of action were described.

The environment of an organisation, whether it be a small group or the community at large, constitutes an external challenge or "normal" stressor. Internal personal reaction to that environment may lead to external action.

A stressor for which the individual is adequately prepared, causes a normal tension, a desire for action. That action may have a constructive aim, but something in the exterior world may block a potentially useful result, rendering that person's effort useless or harmless, but if repeated personal attempts to be useful are continually frustrated, destructive behaviour will be directed against others, or against the person himself.

Should the challenge be one for which the person is ill prepared, there may be a personal block to the stressor, a conflict between the challenge and that individual's aims. He finds himself to be in a state of discomfort, and though his desire for action may lead to constructive or harmless external action, he may either pursue his own aims, contrary to those of the organisation, and to that extent destructive, or he may suppress his desire for action, so altering his normal behaviour, perhaps to the point of breakdown.

Management clearly has the capacity to design the job, and to select and monitor personnel to make sure that the job is both capable of being done, and being done successfully. The community at large has a duty to provide opportunities for work, and to set norms of behaviour which protect the rights of the individual.

In assisting the person to accept challenge, management bears the responsibility for training the employee to cope. The group to which he belongs can develop conformity, so that concerted effort is possible, while the individual depends to some extent upon his previous education and training.

In order to control or direct individual desire for action, management sets objectives, the group determines sanctions within which action is possible, and the individual can be expected to exercise intelligent control. When an individual becomes uncomfortable, in the sense that his efforts are being frustrated, or that inappropriate demands are being made of him, his manager should be both capable of recognising his condition, and willing to provide help. The group to which the unfortunate man belongs and the total medical team, whether within or outside the organisation, must cooperate with the manager, and his subordinate, to reconcile the latter's needs with those of the organisation.

Should all else fail, the patient may become incapable of work, dependent upon various social services, or in extreme cases, may find himself in conflict with the law.

Such a series of propositions might have been dismissed as facile, but a familiar analogy was obvious. It is often said that people are treated with less care and attention than that lavished upon the complex machines they operate. In some of the discussions leading up to the diagram just described, "stress" and "strain" were used as terms. It was pointed out that an engineer might describe stress and strain in individuals in the following terms :

STRESS OR STRAIN IN ENGINEERING TERMS

LOADING (external) —— STRESS (internal) —— STRAIN (internal) may cause

OVERLOADING — OVERSTRESS — YIELDING (irreversible strain) which may not yet prevent function

BREAKDOWN or RUPTURE

Frequent repetition of stress and strain may produce FATIGUE which can then produce RUPTURE without a phase of OVER-LOADING.

In suggesting those agencies who might intervene to prevent undue stress and breakdown, it became clear that, true to the earlier prediction, doctors present were claiming exclusive responsibility for the mental state of people. Others in the group were able to accept this claim only in cases which had already reached breakdown. The doctors were even more upset to learn that trades unions regarded themselves as being the appropriate source of help, and moreover, it was pointed out that very many people in need would not seek help or expect to receive it from doctors, whether at work or at home !

2

Hector the Hedgehog

THE most engaging character in the Windsor seminar emerged as an allegorical figure to illustrate most of what will be reviewed in this book. Someone had suggested that stress in industry was so totally new an experience, that man was no more equipped to deal with it than a hedgehog was equipped to deal with an approaching motor car. From this somewhat flippant remark, Hector the Hedgehog developed. Most people will find it easy to identify themselves with his predicament, in which his natural reaction is to react in a pricklish way to external stressors, while yet having to walk a tightrope with acrobatic skill, carrying a load largely determined by other people.

The tightrope represents the individual's resilience in the face of all the factors with which he has to contend, in the environment in which he finds himself. It will to some extent be determined by himself, though others contribute in forming his attitudes, resources, and spirit. As an adult he derives or maintains support from others he chooses to have about him, such as his family or colleagues, and from the satisfaction he obtains from the activities in which he is engaged at work or at home.

The load Hector carries is in a suitcase, and until he picks it up as he sets out across the abyss, he may not be aware of the burden he is accepting. Indeed, like Hector, we too may be handed a suitcase we do not want but are coerced by others to accept.

Off Hector goes towards his destination. If the tightrope of his ability to cope is not unduly stretched he will confidently balance his way across, but if he senses that his suitcase or his own weight is too great, he will be distracted in his delicate balancing act. If he hears strands of the tightrope snapping, he will become very

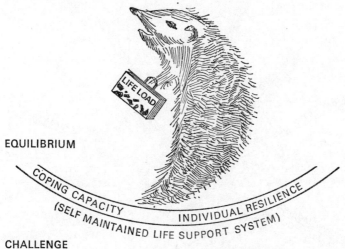

EQUILIBRIUM

COPING CAPACITY
(SELF MAINTAINED LIFE SUPPORT SYSTEM)   INDIVIDUAL RESILIENCE

CHALLENGE

Fig. I Balance Maintained

COPING CAPACITY
THRESHOLD LEVEL
TEMPORARY
BREAKDOWN

EQUILIBRIUM

CHALLENGE

COPING CAPACITY
THRESHOLD LEVEL

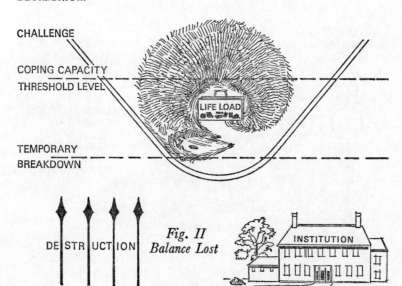

TEMPORARY
BREAKDOWN

DE STR UCT ION

*Fig. II
Balance Lost*

INSTITUTION

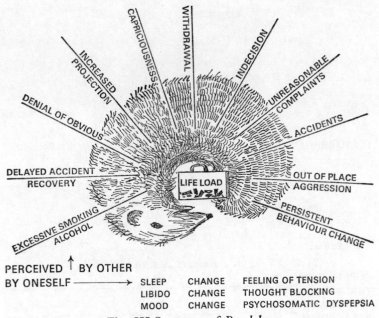

PERCEIVED ↑ BY OTHER
BY ONESELF ⟶

SLEEP	CHANGE	FEELING OF TENSION
LIBIDO	CHANGE	THOUGHT BLOCKING
MOOD	CHANGE	PSYCHOSOMATIC DYSPEPSIA

Fig. III Symptoms of Breakdown

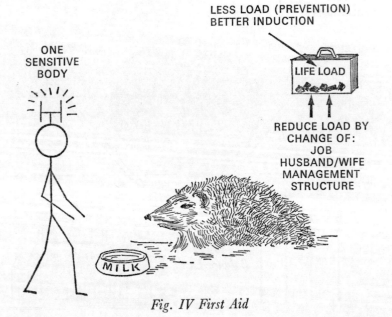

Fig. IV First Aid

anxious, and if the rope stretches too far, the gradient before him becomes too steep to climb. Stuck in the middle of his act, he becomes fearful, adopts instinctive reactions and rolls himself up into a prickly ball, gripping his suitcase to his chest in fright.

Once curled up out on the wire, Hector presents a problem to the rescuer, who has first to approach him, and secondly to coax him to uncurl before anything can be done to get him out of his difficulty. It is to be hoped that help arrives before the rope has stretched beyond the temporary breakdown level, for if he has been suspended below this for too long, his nerve may have gone for good, and he may never be able to regain his former capability. Though perhaps not permanently in an institution, he has become a permanent invalid. If no help comes at all, he may fall to destruction.

If we look more closely at Hector when he is rolled up, we can recognise, label and relate to ourselves many of his prickles. Recourse to greater drinking or smoking are such commonplace reactions to challenge as to need no further comment. The mental turmoil may be so great that normal processes of objective logical thought are lost to the point of denying the obvious. An extension of this is to deny personal responsibility for events, always blaming "them" or "things being as they are" for events. Loss of concentration is followed by an inability to make up his mind, and thus inability to choose an option is further complicated by erratic behaviour in emotional terms, so that at one moment he appears pleased, at another angry, for no obvious reason.

He may become more sensitive to petty irritation, so that he objects frequently about a multitude of things formerly too petty to remark upon. His irritation may lead him to be impatient and to take risks while driving, or at his machine. If he suffers injury as a result, the thought of return to the intolerable situation leads him to delay his resumption of normal work. Alternatively, irritability may lead to out of place aggression, so that a subordinate is harshly or unjustly punished, a child slapped for nothing, or a door slammed. If any of these prickles are not to be found, someone will be able to discover the one marked "persistent behaviour change" because the concept has become part of our language, "He is not himself".

He may also daydream, or explicitly withdraw from a situation which he might previously have tackled, so that now he "wants to have nothing to do with it". He may cheat to cover up less piece work, or produce shoddy goods which have to be scrapped.

Still relating Hector to a human counterpart, it may be that these prickles are present but less obvious just before he has curled up, and when he is still bravely putting on a bold face in a bad situation. He will know that something is wrong. His sleep pattern changes, so that perhaps he cannot get to sleep, or wakes up frequently, or wakes in the early hours of the morning and is unable to get back to sleep. His sexual activity may be decreased or increased, to be expressed in some reckless sexual involvement at work. His mood may be depressed and miserable, or he may overcompensate to be excessively good humoured.

Of course he may realise that he is worried, but surprisingly often he is not, but instead suffers thought blockage, either as loss of concentration, or as inability to remember things or to maintain a clear train of thought : more often he presents his mental problems in the physical disguise of psychosomatic diseases such as stomach ulcers.

If these warning signs result in someone coming to his aid, the "milk" of human kindness, (emotional first aid) may coax him to uncurl, sufficiently not only to resume his journey, but to allow someone else to look at what is in the suitcase. Had more care been taken to assess the weight of the suitcase, Hector or others might not have run the risk of overloading it in the first place : alternatively, if Hector had had an opportunity to get into training with that case, rather than to have it unexpectedly thrust upon him, things might have worked better.

The hedgehog might do better with a reduced load in life's suitcase, or by electing to change for a lighter burden in terms of work, or a different marital partner. This last change, of so fundamental a relationship, is not to be considered lightly, for like any other change, breakdown of marriage brings its own problems.

Whatever the lifeload, it will not be displayed to anyone other than somebody who proffers help and is trusted. Hector could not react to any approach unless he chooses to do so. Who is the sensitive individual who comes to help? It is someone who is sensitive to the needs of others, and who is recognised as being so by his fellows. In only a minority of cases will he be a doctor or clergyman; more often he will be a friend, a colleague at work, or sometimes even a chance acquaintance.

These sensitive people do exist, and may even be recognised. More would come forward if there were opportunities for education and mental first aid training. There is no need to restrict such education to managers or shop stewards; everyone would receive training throughout childhood and maturity, but until experience leads to demand and commitment, there is no point in providing a one-way flow of didactic lecturing.

Anyone might be in Hector's shoes, or next to someone else who is. Not only should he now read on . . . he should press others to do so, and join with others to gain the planned experience which is fundamental to effective training.

3

Stress in the Individual

THERE is no satisfactory definition of "stress" in terms of mental health. Attempts to define it either use a mechanical model in which external stress causes strain inside a material, or describe external stressors which cause internal stress. Throughout this book, the second of these models will be used and the word "stress" will always refer to the internal condition of an individual.

It would be a mistake to assume that stress is always harmful. In all living dynamic organisms, some stress is natural, so that the only human completely unstressed is dead! Children know that the effect of gravity on an inverted onion ensures its survival, because without its internal cellular reactions to the external force, the root of the plant will not turn down, nor the stem grow up. Moreover, if the onion were to be subjected to too much "gravity" in a centrifuge, the stem would be unable to bear its own increased weight and would collapse, the delicate plant breaking down more easily than a sturdy one.

In some experiments connected with space research, men have been floated in water at body temperature so that they feel weightless. With eyes and ears covered they see and hear nothing; they breathe air through a mask and feed through a tube, while floating motionless. Within hours they become so confused by the complete absence of external stimuli or stressors (objects or persons causing stress), and lose sense of time and place so much, that one of them has tried to tear the air mask from his face forgetting that his life depends upon it. One could almost describe this reaction as being bored to death.

We can say that a condition of harmful stress may be caused within someone by an abnormal load—too little being as harmful as too much, and the unexpected being potentially more disturbing to the person unprepared or untrained to withstand it. Everyone is aware that "one man's meat is another man's poison", and that what may be a stimulating challenge to one of us might literally drive another "off the rails" of normal rational behaviour.

Even though we cannot define the term "stress", we seem to be able to notice the condition of stress in members of our family, or in our neighbours at home or at work. We go further in recognising something likely to cause stress in one of those individuals even before the event, and sometimes we are aware that the stress is caused by too great a degree or a number of stressors—the last straw—or that the unexpected or unusual event takes someone by surprise. It is therefore important to state what may be obvious, namely that anyone who has read this far is aware that he or she already understands something of the subject covered by this book, and that anyone may suffer or cause harmful stress.

In order to reduce my own anxieties about "he" and "she" I am going to assume from now on that the masculine form covers everyone (that helps me but may well infuriate feminists!).

For some reason, executives are popularly supposed to be those most at risk, and they are assumed to be so because of some factors peculiar to the nature of their responsibilities. This exclusive assumption is open to question. Certainly they are one of the groups of the population more at risk than others, but the factors which combine to cause harmful stress and breakdown in the young or the old are scattered throughout the day, the month, or the year, whether at paid occupations or working at home. The "burned out executive" does not differ fundamentally from the prematurely aged, downtrodden apathetic worker. There is a different significance of their condition for each, particularly the effect of the drop in the standard of living which makes the executive's fall from grace more acutely miserable.

Interference with normal drives and aspirations may cause frustration. "Letting off steam" leads to aggression, or withdrawal from constructive participation in the life of the family, the organisation, or the community at large. The effort spent in coping with the often unnecessary conflicts so aroused must be an enormous waste of the nervous energy which might better be directed to the improvement of the quality of life of all concerned.

It has been suggested that individuals have five levels of need.[1] The physiological necessities of food and drink maintain the life in the organism, while the capacity to reproduce tissue, to heal wounds or sickness and the ability to procreate offspring assures the survival of the species. At a second level, the safety and survival of the individual, particularly when young, in what is basically a hostile environment, depends upon the shelter of a home, and on adequate clothing to protect from extremes of heat, cold, wind and rain.

As these two levels of need are satisfied the developing individual has more opportunities for attention to and from other individuals. Social relationships provide for care and protection in the family, cooperation with others in production or defence, and loyalties to the larger group to which immediate neighbours belong.

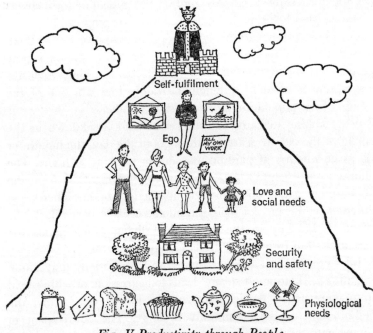

Fig. V Productivity through People

As soon as a group is formed, each individual in it rises to the fourth level of need, and has a sense of his own identity, of what he has to offer, and of what he expects to derive from others in the group. He becomes aware of the part he plays and of the rank to which he believes he is entitled. To some extent and from a variety of sources, he derives self-respect, and if his perception of his role is justified in the view of others, he can achieve the fifth and highest level of satisfaction to be derived from self actualisation, colloquially expressed as "doing one's own thing".

In a study of jobs in several countries, sources of satisfaction were gathered into two main groups.[2] Some are said to be "negative incentives" in that their absence, or deficiency, give rise to an environment which, by being even minimally irritant, affects the quality of work done by distracting some attention of the individual. Such "hygiene factors" if satisfactory contribute to a healthy work situation, but do not themselves constitute a reward. They simply play a part in providing a suitable context in which work can take place.

HYGIENE FACTORS (negative incentives)	MOTIVATORS (positive incentives)
Company Policy and Administration	Achievement
Supervision	Recognition
Relationship with Supervisor	Work Itself
Work Conditions	Responsibility
Salary	Advancement
Relationship with Peers	Growth
Personal Life	
Relationship with Subordinates	
Status	
Security	

The analogy between this list of "hygiene factors" and the more usual concept of hygiene in terms of health is particularly close if one considers, as an example, payment for work. The appetite for a level of remuneration can be satisfied temporarily, but no matter how acceptable the reward for a specific job may be at any one time, that satisfaction will wear off quite independently of other factors like increases in the cost of living, seniority, or productivity. Just as the satisfaction of a good meal gives way inevitably to hunger, so there is a constant need for more pay.

This idea of an inexorable rise in expectation is not new. Indeed it was noticed early in the nineteenth century by a contemporary commentator on the French scene after the Revolution. Speaking of the common people, Alexis de Tocqueville said: "Their condition had never improved so rapidly as in the previous twenty years, and yet they found their position the more intolerable, the better it became." In other words, advance up the scale of needs alters one's attitude to those needs, and adjusts expectations to a higher level than previously was the case.

Positive incentives on the other hand really do motivate the individual. The list of motivators can be said to correspond with the concept of self-actualisation referred to earlier. By recognising the significance of five levels of need, the objectives of the group or organisations can be reconciled with those of the people who make up its parts. The "stick and carrot" approach only punishes, or rewards. By offering an opportunity for satisfaction after having dealt with the hygiene factors in the environment, individual drive may be reconciled to the objectives of the group and harnessed to them, instead of frequently diverging from, or even actually opposing, them.

While there is little, if any, denial of the validity of the basic drives, or the motivation of people, there are objections to their practical application. It is assumed not to be practical to suggest changing or scrapping enormously expensive production lines which are the cheapest way to produce the goods demanded by a consumer society. The sequence of stages in manufacture has been a major factor in the organisation of the labour force required to operate the machines; the processes themselves may be potentially or actually dangerous to those working at them. But opportunities do arise to question these basic assumptions.

Philips Electrical Industries have altered the structure of work groups making television sets, so that small groups of workers have responsibility to indent for their own stores and each member of that group makes a complete television set and acts as his or her own quality control. Even the classical example of the Ford motor production line, long quoted as being an inevitable feature of mass production, is now the subject of question. Volvo Motors in Sweden[3] are about to produce cars in a sequence which takes due note of human need, rather than perpetuate the traditional system of adapting human beings to machines in new factories. (If this Swedish experiment works, it will be an irony that the historical significance of Henry Ford's ideas themselves become "bunk", just as he dismissed those historical events which he considered had no significance to the present.)

The conflict assumed to exist only between organisational needs and those of people are not confined to industrial situations. Roughly speaking, for every man who repeats a monotonous task, whether manual or clerical, there is a woman who repeatedly dusts, sweeps, and makes beds for no pay; for every man cut off from his fellow workers by distance or noise, there is a woman isolated in her kitchen in a dormitory suburb; and the housewife is often more at risk from burns, scalds, electrocution, falls and other accidents than her husband who may have less concern for her welfare and safety in practice than he believes his employer has for him. Should anyone question that rather sweeping statement, let him reflect that it is the women's journals and consumer associations which complain about the quality and safety of the machines that husbands design, produce, market and sell. If you find even that thought unacceptable, further reflection might lead you to doubt the justice of compensation for so called "industrial" injury, when the housewife who falls down stairs in her own home while doing her own work gets nothing but sympathy, if that!

In summary then, throughout his life the human animal requires physiological and psychological stimuli from outside to promote and maintain internal activity. That activity may turn into a stress reaction either as a result of exposure to the few forces which are harmful in themselves, or more often as a result of the intensity of otherwise normal stimuli which are set at intolerable levels.

At present, material needs related to pay and salaries form the particular point of conflict in most industrial disputes. Growing awareness of emotional needs, and appreciation of their magnitude, has led to the study of how they might be satisfied. Many professions are concerned with the signs that indicate lack of satisfaction, and with the treatment or even prevention of this deficiency. The remedies suggested depend upon the viewpoint of the commentator who may regard the answer to be related to health, or to productivity, or to the contentment of the individual. It is noteworthy that the various professions or organisations carrying out studies from these differing viewpoints do not always collaborate or even communicate their ideas to each other. Doctors, in particular, even have ethical rules designed to prevent them communicating in individual cases; these rules are often interpreted as absolving the doctor from making any general comment about the patient's situation at all.

Many other lists of emotional satisfactions have been prepared in addition to those I have already quoted, but there is general agreement on three basic needs :

> Membership of a group
> Individual fulfilment
> Shared responsibility

These are derived from the nature of the work, or from one's companions, or from both. The degree to which these needs are satisfied varies between individuals, and within the same individual at different times, ages, or circumstances. Understanding of those needs and conscious control may help individuals to find new sources of satisfaction if and when old ones are lost, but to teach that understanding and control takes a long time and the individual being taught may be too old to learn, or perhaps cannot be helped before it is too late.

Without these basic satisfactions, wasteful or even dangerous reactions may occur either externally in the shape of personal or social antagonisms, ("letting off steam", "taking it out on someone") or internally by setting up vicious circles of personal frustration, psychological and even physical ill health, which in turn cause a greater sense of frustration and so on. Observations in many parts of the world show that these signs increase as countries become rapidly industrialised. As a society becomes industrialised the opportunities for satisfaction at work become fewer and leisure activities seldom provide adequate compensation.

Besides the denial of satisfaction, other forces cause stress in individuals or groups, and these forces are becoming more numerous and stronger. It is not hard to see that over-population and capacity for destruction are increasing daily. The dangers of the first are not just shortage of food : the threat to individual territory is probably more likely to lead a man to destructive irrational behaviour if we are to judge from animal studies. If this destructive tendency is inherited by man from his pre-human carnivorous ancestors, he may well revert to it in overwhelming force under extreme stress. Restraints to violence are less since the ethical or religious codes which inhibited destruction are weaker. Social habits permit or even encourage violence, in some cases for its own sake, since the approval of the group to which one belongs may overrule personal values and inhibitions against the use of violence.

Justifiable brutality and "judicial" interrogation and torture are coming back, while race prejudice provides an easy and permanent channel for the release of destructive forces which is sanctioned by the immediate group.

Industrial problems must be seen in the context of such individual or community attitudes, which certainly affect behaviour at work. Both management and workers need to be concerned with social pressures and behaviour, and greater understanding will only come as a result of better collaboration and more open communication between all the professions and disciplines interested in human behaviour within industry or outside it.

If mental health is the state of equilibrium between the many stressors, that state when disturbed may rapidly readjust if the individual's internal stress is not too great to allow him to do so. But the equilibrium may be upset to the point of breakdown or even death. Neither the stressors nor the reactions to them are constant, and elsewhere in this book the dynamic process of repeated adjustment will be emphasised. The reactions may be literally unconscious, in the sense that the individual may not be aware that he is suffering stress.

If unnoticed, stress may be outside intelligent control either by the individual himself, or anyone else, though even the unconscious control by that individual may be adequate and successful.

If we are aware of our reactions, and unless we deny that human beings should take responsibility for their actions, we have a duty to consider whether our own reaction in stressful situations is beneficial or harmless, dangerous to ourselves or to others, now or later. If we are aware that it is dangerous, we must try to prevent this reaction, or at least attempt to minimise the damage.

Doctors are traditionally and naturally concerned in the breakdown of physical or mental health, which may possibly lead through depression to suicide or a fatal illness. Early signs of the stage of breakdown are all those chronic neurotic and psychosomatic illnesses which are recorded in increasing numbers in most industrialised or developing countries. Together with other types of illness caused by the individual's own misguided efforts to deal with tension and stress by drink and drugs including tobacco, these minor complaints may be indications that the individual is approaching breakdown. Add to these, accidents occurring on roads, in factories, or at home, and we have a list of results of someone's unresolved tensions, diminished judgement, and loss of control which may bring the patient into the hands of the physician, surgeon, psychiatrist or even undertaker!

Such sequels of lost equilibrium are only marginally the concern of the medical profession. The individual may attack others, verbally or physically, or provoke others to attack him. He may be arrested by the police as a criminal, or be so effective in his behaviour that the police do not catch him. Many sequels do no harm to anyone, as in sport or hobbies, or better still benefit other people as well as the man concerned, when they are expressed as better work, social reform or creative art, music and architecture.

It is important to realise that groups behave in ways comparable to those of individuals, to the point that breakdown of group health may occur. Relations deteriorate, suspicion and open antagonisms grow, and group violence may erupt. Alternatively, the group, like the individual, may choose harmless or constructive activity as an outlet for its stress. When groups react to stressors and express their internal stress in constructive or destructive way, they do not necessarily come to the attention of the doctor. But industrialists, and social scientists do study these reactions, and since doctors themselves form a group, they too

LET THE HUNGRY MAKE YOUR MONEY GROW.

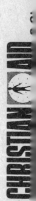

Most of us now spend nearly a quarter of our income on food. That's one thing inflation has done to us. So you might decide that this Christian Aid Week you can't help the world's hungry.

But before you make that decision, think for a moment what inflation has done to people in the poorest countries – where they were much worse off to start with.

In Ghana (West Africa) food prices rose 20 per cent last year, and families there have to spend HALF their earnings on food.

In Bangladesh it's worse. Rice and cooking oil prices have both increased six-fold, and sugar seven-fold. A farm worker there needs to spend a full day's wage (24p) to buy enough rice to feed his family for one day. Or let them go hungry.

Money raised in Christian Aid Week is not used to buy food at inflationary prices, but on development schemes which help the hungry and the poor to raise food production or to learn a wage-earning trade.

They do all the work; we provide some of the money. And money never works harder than when put into the hands of the poor. Their lives depend on it. They'll make your gift of money grow.

So please give what you can reasonably afford. Thank you.

CHRISTIAN AID

have an interest in group behaviour, though it is outside the performance of their traditional role.

Before the stage of breakdown just described is reached, there is a stage of disturbed equilibrium which certainly can be recognised. Most people can notice in their friends, without formulating what the matter is, that he is tense, irritable, "under the weather" or "not himself." Of those who are aware of such changes in their neighbour, many go further to accept their responsibility for help and offer first aid without realising exactly what they are doing, but nevertheless being very successful. This "first aid" is part of the professional experience of many people, such as personnel managers, clergy and social workers, but they have no monopoly. Parents do it to their children who in turn display it towards their parents. This two-way flow of help is often not noticed or recognised, but it is there, and extends beyond family boundaries. If managers provide help for their juniors, so do some subordinates provide help for their seniors—personal secretaries are obvious examples. No doubt many breakdowns have been, and many more will be, saved—often in complete ignorance that anyone was at risk at all, and therefore without invoking medical aid. Others have not been saved, and tragedies have occurred.

The factors which determine the choice of reaction can be grouped as external and internal, though it is always their interplay which matters. The interaction of various factors within individuals or groups are all the time changing, and several factors in different areas may act together. We must not only consider the obvious threat, but all the other factors in the situation, including the help available from superiors, peers, and subordinates. It is more often the total weight of minor stresses which produces breakdown than an intense specific stressor.

The internal factors include the person's constitution and heredity, and his previous upbringing or education in its widest sense. One person may be more inclined to conform to the demands of his own peer group; another to rebel against dictatorial authority; another responds to appeals which play on his image of himself as a social reformer: while another may be jealous of his status. If these factors are recognised and understood, "first aid" at this pre-breakdown phase can be more effective.

Unfortunately, the underlying causes of behaviour are taught too little and those concerned have to learn as they go along. Interest seems to be confined to particular roles or people, so that when helpers attempt to act, there is a need to explain to the "victim" being helped what the motives of the helpers are, lest he suspect that he is being "manipulated" for sinister reasons. Doctors in most circumstances are assumed to be trustworthy, but are viewed with suspicion when working in this field in industry. Nevertheless the practical difficulties, and the theoretical possibilities, of what doctors have to offer both "sides" of industry deserve attention.

A stage which occurs even before those just described, is both more difficult to recognise, and much more difficult to control. For instance, fear does occur in danger, but physical reaction may be mastered by training. This approach to the inevitable fear expected in military operations is seldom appropriate in industry, where there may be time, or it may be easier or more expedient to remedy the ill effect of any stressor rather than to aim to prevent it. The whole point of education and training is to alter or modify the individual before the impact of the stressor. Otherwise we may be confined to helping the individual to pick up the pieces after his breakdown.

If the individual's tendencies are understood so that he can be helped, how much better it would be if they could be modified so that he does not need help at all. This has been the aim of many educators of particular groups, and with some success. With the possible exception of Dr. Spock and child guidance experts, surprisingly few doctors have seen it as their job until this last decade. While sex education has become widespread and First Aid for injuries is beginning to be taught in junior schools, "education for life" is only being talked about.

Doctors do not have the prime responsibility for public attention to mental health, but other professions such as educators, and in industry the managers and trade unionists, do. While doctors in industry have some special problems to overcome in winning trust, all doctors have a part to play and could collaborate much more with both management and trade unions in the care of their patients, or the maintenance of group health.

As a profession, doctors should at least communicate their knowledge and their skills. After all, they see the breakdowns, and their competence in dealing with them may assist them in convincing others, from whom in turn the doctors have much to learn. The doctor could more often act as a bridge between other professions involved, so that all can understand their antagonisms, and resolve their hostility. Social psychologists and animal ethologists have something to say on group behaviour, inherited tendencies, and on stress.

In brief, we are in a position where there is more pressure, more aggression aroused, but less outlet available in work or leisure. There is less stabilising force to control its direction and more tendencies which encourage it to set up vicious circles of destruction with increased power to destroy. Greater understanding demands better education which may lead to more control, and all those concerned need to collaborate. Industry has the means and the money to take a lead. If by debasing the satisfactions of work, industry in the last century has increased tension, it has a responsibility now to try to reverse the trend. To some extent, schemes for retraining those whose jobs have become obsolete are a start in this direction.

Not only are employers challenged. Unions and workers' associations themselves may be as obsessed by money as any employer at whom they point an accusing finger. How often does a union demand danger money instead of adequate protection for its members? Why do union negotiators mean "fewer hours at basic pay" when they refer to a reduction in the working week? Why does a union appear to condone almost ruthless lack of regard for fellow workers by powerful sectional interests within its own membership?

4

Stress in the Organisation

BECAUSE of the varied adaptability and resilience of each person in an organisation, it is misleading to think of factors like time pressure, monotony, or conflicting demands as being necessarily "stress". It is easier to think of situations which may or may not include some of those factors, as being ones in which the individual is at risk, or as circumstances which predispose to, but do not inevitably produce, partial or complete breakdown of the internal personal equilibrium which has been described. The pattern of the stress produced will be determined both by the external forces, and by the internal stress state of the person affected, and that composite pattern will determine the reaction as a mood change, an anxiety state, or more serious mental or physical disease.

The exterior stress producing forces are balanced in a dynamic system by individual internal resistance, but this balance is much more complex than a simple "see-saw". Rather than merely balancing two ends of a plank on a central bar, the problem is more like trying to balance a circular plate on a needle point. Several forces are at work, such as the "moral support" that may be derived from one's fellows, which boosts one's internal capacity to resist—at least for a time. An individual, his groups, the organisation in which he works, and the environment in which the organisation functions can act independently or jointly on one another. In considering factors which may cause stress, there are constants and variables.

The compensatory and behavioural changes possible inside a living organism provide a much greater capacity for stress than the strength of the materials of which it is made. Compensation may continue until the cause of stress passes and the stress itself is relieved. But the stressor causes breakdown when it exceeds that load to which the individual or the organisation can adapt. However a system already actively compensating under load is less likely to have the capacity to respond to new stresses which it may encounter. Death of the individual may well be a most tragic outcome of the failure of compensation. So it is the compensated states which need to be identified because those in whom they occur are at risk. If it is an organisation which is being considered in this light, the equivalent of individual disease and death may be the decline and disintegration of the organisation. Just as the individual may present his stress to his doctor in terms of illness or symptoms, so may the organisation display disguised abnormality, or cause some of the individuals who are its constituent parts to present as if they were personally ill. While this is a gross over-simplification of a very complex process, it may convey the idea that behaviour is the result of a whole lot of processes at work, a system within a system.

As a piece of a larger organism, the individual may be considered as seeking out a niche, an environment which provides for him a balance between sufficient satisfaction and reward and the minimum of stress and discomfort. The description of what has happened is made after the event, which may not have been the result of a conscious effort on a man's part. Indeed it is often true that he does not find a niche so much as gravitates, or even is nudged into one, but whatever the process, many men are likely to be found existing in states of equilibrium in which work load and emotional satisfaction are in balance.

When the environment or any other force enforces a change in one side of the balance, at least an attempt at adjustment follows. It is at this point that individuals are at risk. Adaptation may be easy enough, but if it cannot be achieved detectable strain may ensue with eventual breakdown. Peculiar gratifications and hidden satisfactions are sometimes revealed when compassionate efforts are made to ameliorate working conditions, or when a compliment is expressed by promotion, without due regard to the capability of the individual being so "rewarded". The so called "Peter principle" is another way of stating this.[4] ("Peter's Principle" is the doctrine which states that most large businesses have as their unspoken career planning philosophy, perhaps without realising it, the approach that a man is promoted until he reaches his "level of incompetence.")

Most work involves group activities, and certainly membership of an organisation does. Naturally occurring "work group" activity will emerge where a group tackles a task and divides labour appropriately between individual capacities and the activities needed to complete the task. But groups will be motivated by other functions than the work itself. These may emerge with great intensity or be initiated when change is thrust on a group. Leadership conflicts are more likely to be revealed as group responses than as obvious competition or open animosity between the "contenders for the title". It is perhaps because complex group behaviour is disturbingly unconscious and apparently irrational that there is a reluctance to look closely at group dynamics in live industrial situations. It might be a valuable principle of change if the group dynamics existing before the stressful situation happened were uncovered and compared with those that may follow the event, or sometimes even only the threat of change.

Individuals within an organisation must be affected by the changes occurring within that organisation as it adapts to the pressures that historical change produces. They are not exempt even when it elects to resist change. For if it resists successfully for a long time it runs the risk of eventual extinction or of having to respond to catastrophic change. Some, at least, of its members, alert to these impending dangers, will be under stress made worse possibly by their impotence to do much about events. This is another manifestation of a system within a system.

A list of stressor situations, descending from the organisation's end down to personal idiosyncrasy, can be prepared but this order is apparent rather than real, because in a dynamic system significant changes can go in any direction, and need not necessarily go up or down through each stage.

1. Stress in individuals due to changes facing an organisation

from its environment (and progress towards institutionalis-
ation).

2. Stress in individuals arising from their change or development within an organisation. (This includes normal advancement, projection system, interpersonal clashes, and
   moral issues.)
3. Stress from an individual's group relations, either with his
   family, or as real or imagined disloyalty to earlier working
   groups.
4. Stress from specifically individual factors.

Such a ranking is incomplete, but the list does provide a framework against which "organisation versus individual" conflict can
be considered.

In a model similar to that representing five levels of individual
need, the environment might be regarded as having four levels
of complexity.

The lowest could be considered as a flat surface upon which
"good" or "bad" things—or "organisms"—were distributed at
random. A lone organism wandering about that plain might
easily avoid the bad, and approach the good. At the second level
of complexity, the good and bad heaps are clustered in such a
way that to get to the good things, the bad have to be overcome
or endured, rather than merely avoided as before. At the third
level, one adds to this pattern of clusters more organisms, each of
which has to regard all the others as additional obstacles or
impediments to reaching the "good" heaps and each organism
has to determine not only whether to accept short term discomfort
for longer term gain, but whether to come to terms with another
organism so that both can survive rather than fight to the death
unnecessarily.

To those three levels of complexity Emery and Trist[5] added
a fourth. Suppose that the clustered "good" and "bad" heaps
are placed not on a flat static plain, but upon a surface ran-
domly moving in all dimensions, so that there is lateral movement
of the ground, and alternating heights or hollows in the same place.
On this shifting ground, which is like a sheet blowing in the wind,
the organisms who are developing some love-hate relationships

have to compete with each other, and find the "good" and the "bad", with little help from fixed points of reference, and with great difficulty in maintaining their own balance. The number and intensity of stimuli may now begin to cause stress within the individuals, or cause improvement or breakdown of the relationship between the individual organisms which make up the organised society, or the number of organised societies, inhabiting the turbulent environment. It is clear then that organisations have their stresses, and that their survival cannot be taken for granted when looking at the disturbed behaviour of individuals within them. As an organisation grows and moves towards becoming an institution, there are changes that occur within it which might parallel either the biological loss of the polymorphous capacity of cells to develop in a number of directions, or the fixation of structures and functions that happen within an increasingly complex and sophisticated organism. In other words logistic problems develop. More complex communications are needed, but more can therefore go astray. More diverse roles are needed, to operate the system; hence more chance of confusion and frustration if things go wrong.

One of the most common stressors acting upon individuals is change. One aspect of change in the organisation has already been referred to, and another is the increase in that rate of change due to the rapidity of technological advance. The environment or its demands may change faster than the capacity of the organisation to adapt to them. This introduces degrees of uncertainty which need to be dealt with in a way quite unlike the response to simpler environments of earlier times, or of less industrialised countries.

In terms of the individual as part of the organisation, his own advancement may alter the demands upon him, and examples of this will appear later. Meanwhile a commercial organisation has to respond to technological changes and may even have to change totally its products or services if it is to survive. Therefore the individuals within it may need to adapt to new things, and learn or develop entirely new skills. The progress of a man up through an organisation, especially if he moves from a craft or specialist function to an administrative and managerial one, may cause him to be confronted with a need for skills for which he has had no training whatever. In such a situation, motivation is critical. If "a field marshal's baton is burning in his knapsack" his own drive to succeed will overcome many of these difficulties. If, however, he is promoted reluctantly his morale may suffer in the face of them. Apparently straightforward progress upward is not stress-free. Even the tycoon, the man who has the drive and capacity to make a great deal of money very quickly, may find himself totally unable to make the change to manage the organisation that he has developed, as it increases in size from his own capacity to make money and expand.

"Projection System" is a convenient term which refers to a number of "them and us" situations, where changes are compelled by changing times. When one company amalgamates with, or is taken over by another, then there are loyalty and identity problems. The man who believes that "the Wogs begin at Calais" is not going to find international or transcultural co-operation easy. There are bound to be problems when giants like, for example, Dunlop and Pirelli merge, and these problems are quite different from the expansion by a company from one country into another.

Individuals and groups grow used to traditional rivals and enemies, but if for example "the unions" are felt to become identified with "the bosses", as in some recent disputes, then there are at least agitations to reform the traditional pattern. Demarcation disputes are part of this, and are even more insidious when they are referred to as "specialist problems".

Specialist groups, moreover, tend to arrogate to themselves exclusive powers and rights of membership. Many doctors seem to believe that they are the only ones who have had that laying on of hands which gives them the right and the power to heal the sick. A system which needs great freedom of action and role versatility for its most effective and economical functioning is felt as a threat by such specialist groups, leading to demarcation disputes or rivalries and resistances which, although apparently petty, are enormously crippling for efficiency.

Inter-personal clashes between people who are either temporarily or permanently incompatible are common and need little further explanation, except to say that what is perceived to be "true", is much more important than the truth itself.

"Moral issues" are a major area of potential stress. Possibly this is not so for many because our consciences and scruples may be the most adaptable parts of our personalities. Possibly strong and rigid individuals resign or withdraw, the expedient yield and the weak suffer a bad conscience. Unfortunately not only the rigid but the paranoid also resign. There is a whole area of moral issues at stake in the whole tenor of business, and not only in the sense of competition and advantage seeking and taking. If profit, as opposed to service, is the dominant motive (and it is very easy to argue that it must be) then a further area of conflict may be introduced.

There can be an internal conflict in an individual between his own ethos, and the ethos of the organisation of which he is part. The salesman expected to sell aggressively something for which he has no regard; the manager expected to hire and fire in circumstances which he does not consider appropriate; the doctor who must abort a woman because it is in his contract to do so, whatever his own conviction : this type of internal conflict is far more widespread than is generally thought. These and several other stressors could be regarded as the "toxicity" of the management situation.

There are several classical examples of this complex picture the foregoing paragraphs have attempted to convey. The armed services, or the Church, are archetypes of the institution. The institutional Church is up to the neck in adaptation problems. It has progressively become an hierarchical institution which has responded to historical demands and has, in turn, contributed to historical changes with an expediency much more appropriate to the service of Mammon than to the witness of its declared Lord. Though at present maladapted to needs and bogged down in trappings, the capacity for survival of such bodies must not be underestimated.

Those who were "called" into service were called to something which perhaps seems to change faster than they can adapt. Those men concerned most with the Church's message still find ways to proclaim it, and are likely to be in dispute only with those who wish to change the message as their form of adaptation. But some were attracted to the institution primarily because it had atmosphere and ambience. It had theatre. It had status. It had a dependent flock. To some such men the changes have proved very disturbing. There is no question that there have been feelings of futility and a sense of frustration in many clerics which has hitherto either led only to heart searching or to low morale. There is still theatre and some develop this. Others follow a vogue for pastoral counselling to restore a sense of purpose, of mission once again.

The consumer's expectations have a relevance of their own, and it may be an extra problem for the clergy to meet consumers' expectations when their own views have suffered such change. One of the phenomena which we now see is that of the resurgence of protest in the mediaeval sense, by which the consumer introduces yet another force to which adaptation has to be made by the clergy.

It is really quite amazing how much resistance to change is possible within an institution and how irrational—apparently—and how regressive resistance can be : a fact usually overlooked entirely when Utopian ideas for change are in the air.

In the Army where technology is continuously changing, and often very up to date, many of the social systems remain unchanged to the point of being anachronistic. There are many other fields where changing demands do leave organisations like stranded whales. Three examples are the entertainment industry, the railways and the Co-operative movement. Some, like the entertainment industry, have suffered successive waves of change with fresh uncertainty from each. Specialist and not very adaptable groups like cinema and theatre musicians, have had their normal pattern of life ended abruptly. Inevitable changes enforced on us from without do create groups at risk, but not all the individuals suffer stress, let alone break down. Sensitive measures of increased risk and increased potential morbidity have yet to be quantified, and are likely to be behavioural measures rather than ones couched in terms of pathological change.

A very important area of risk centres around marriage and the family. Many men who are successful in industry are faced with major problems in that their degree of personal involvement in their organisation will change as they progress and have greater responsibility. Their personal freedom may well diminish. Regular hours of work become a thing of the past and unexpected, but not always unwelcome, separations from home may occur. Temptations or the arousal of jealousies which threaten stability of a marriage and family may well follow. Again, a successful man may rise in social status but have a wife who is unable or unwilling to "move up" with him, and who then feels utterly lost in unfamiliar surroundings. The man himself may, of course, respond by feeling either an outcast from his old group or over compensate, so that many men with undoubted ability drop back or refuse to budge because they cannot face the challenge.

The realisation of having reached one's ceiling may be a considerable problem, and may provoke the depression by which the crisis is clinically presented. This point in one's career may coincide with the climacteric, which exists in men as well as women, who are then "one degree under" before the new exterior stressor is applied.

Individual factors include not just stability and adaptability, enormously important as they are, but inborn factors like intelligence and attributes like Hudson's "convergers and divergers"[6] which influence a man's potential for meeting new demands.

Doctors, especially those working in hospital, are interested in, and react to, disease and pathology. It is important to present and reinforce the opposite concept, that of still healthy groups and individuals at risk with no pathology yet involved. One management task ought to be to try to minimise if possible the incidence of stress. Much can be done by attempting to predict what events and reactions will follow the introduction of change. If individual breakdown has already occurred, it may be important for the doctor to comment about management issues, the patient's or management's style, and confusion with roles, because these are often an important part of the patient's total problem. Though clinically trained, and though it may not have entered their heads that preservation of mental health should be part of their motivation, doctors in industry must contribute to prediction of stress as part of their management function. They can then have a purpose in forward planning, not just one of binding up wounds.

The appropriate roles for doctors in an industrial society and the good or bad effects of different sorts of industrial experience, deserve further study by both management and doctors. Modern accounting procedure has moved from book-keeping and auditing to the development of techniques for the anticipation of future states, with a consequent much greater control of affairs by means of predictive measures like cash flow analysis and forms of budgetary control. Ideally we should attempt to move in this direction with human predictions.

The major obstacle is the identification and measurement of human behaviour resulting from an enormous number of variables, which are much more difficult to observe than financial phenomena. However, some of the more "toxic" factors in management can be identified now, and remedies suggested. What is more, greater sensitivity and insight may lead to recognition of the disturbed, but still compensated, states.

5

Stress in Management

THE theme of this book is to persuade the reader that whoever he is he has a part to play in the promotion and maintenance of mental health. This chapter may help those to whom some of the situations described in theory are already familiar in practice, and help them to derive confidence from the realisation that perhaps their appreciation of a situation, which they may have no opportunity to discuss elsewhere, was correct.

The situations described occur widely not only in industry but also in many other areas. Indeed it is a pity that we have not yet become accustomed to the idea that each of us has an occupation, paid or not, formal or otherwise, and that situations like those referred to in an industrial management setting occur wherever any one person co-operates, interacts, or works with another.

The factors which create stress in conventional management situations are described here without any attempt to interpret them in medical or psychological terms.

In the management of a large complex organisation, stress is inevitable. The whole process of management is essentially the art and science of identifying conflicting variables to best advantage, and if that reconciliation of conflict is an integral part of a job then that job must be stressful. However, successful people in the field of management are well able to accommodate stress in large quantities. Problems only arise where an individual is stretched beyond his capacity for stress, or where an unsuitable person finds himself in a role with which he cannot cope.

The latter point is a special problem, and this chapter confines itself to the situation in which a man who is temperamentally suited to a management role may nevertheless find himself in circumstances which he finds intolerable. Intolerable situations may arise in two main ways. First where the number or dimension of the stressors rise beyond the normal level; or, secondly, where there are abnormal stress situations which raise the total stress burden beyond that individual's capacity.

It has become fashionable in recent years to present in more systematic form the obligation of a manager to achieve results. In expressing this in terms of objectives there is a benefit to the manager, in that the establishment of clear personal objectives does tend to eradicate the fears of a man who does not know what is expected of him. Objectives can eliminate undesirable tensions, but at the same time, management by objectives puts people under the strain of knowing that they have an obligation to do certain things against a time deadline and on a basis against which they can be measured and assessed. This form of pressure has always been there, though perhaps less readily discernible than it is today, but the nature of the pressure has changed.

The subordinate may find himself in a situation in which he has helped to set a target which he has been subtly and perhaps unconsciously persuaded to agree is reasonable. If that target is not reached in the time allowed, his contribution to setting that target may be interpreted by the superior as a sign of the subordinate's poor judgement. Thus, in addition to being under scrutiny from above, the subordinate runs a risk of being scrupulously critical of his own performance, so that an objective which for any reason drifts out of reach is not discarded though the unfortunate subordinate knows sometimes well in advance, that he cannot reach it.

The acceptable standard of management performance is steadily and inexorably increasing, so that the manager who manages to keep up with last year's standards, may, if he is failing to learn new things and keep up to date, be starting to fall below steadily rising standards of acceptable performance. The "traditional" type of older manager has to learn a new philosophy of appraisal, let alone a possibly complex system which expresses that philosophy. In addition to reacting to what is happening, he has to learn to interpret new information presented in a new format, in order to predict what may happen in the future. To use a military analogy, he is expected to abandon the secure position from which he can fire when "he sees the whites of the enemies' eyes", and to go out to search for and deal with threats which may materialise unexpectedly or not at all.

Most managers find that there is more demand for their time and resources than they are able to meet, and they are therefore constantly faced with demands in excess of the supply of resources. This is stressful in terms of pressure on managers' personal time. As well as resolving conflict between competing demands for limited resources, they have to cope with conflicting demands upon themselves. The classic example of this is the manager who has to answer frequent queries which are a distraction to his attempts to do his own work. How many such people look forward to the end of the day because "everyone else has gone and now I can do some work"? How often is that extended into the family's time, when a man has to take his briefcase home to "read the literature" at the weekend?

A factor which adds to the problems of a man in a fast-moving, high-pressure business is that of fatigue, since a great deal of business travelling is done outside normal working time. To commuting can be added the problems of driving in traffic and over longer distances; the difficulties encountered in crossing time zones on long distance flights; strange beds in hotels; the excessive food and drink that tends to be the pattern of hospitality; and boredom on business trips.

It is a normal part of the management theme that a man is under pressure to produce results at a predetermined cost, to have restrictions on the amount of money he can spend in particular ways, and to have conflicting demands for limited financial resources, so that the financial constraints of the organisation add to the burden of the manager who has results to achieve.

Many managers find that the demands of their job conflict with the demands of their family and that, in today's world, it is unfortunately all too often the family demands that are neglected. This can cause stress in the home environment and create antipathy in the home towards the manager's job. In that situation "daddy" is rarely at home to greet the children when they come home from school. Sometimes it is in the interests of "daddy's job" rather than those of the child that he or she is

packed off to boarding school, with perhaps only limited acceptance by the mother of the resulting deprivation of her children.

Managers live in a competitive environment where, if you are
not going forward you are going back, and where the socially
respectable ethic is to be ambitious for oneself seeking promotion
and advancement, and to be constantly considering career aspirations in relation to opportunities. One of the most unhappy
people which our present industrial system tends to produce is
the man who has aspirations, or whose wife has aspirations for
him, which are in excess of his talents. The frustrations and
damage to dignity which stems from a man failing to achieve his
own ambitions adds stress. Appraisal systems originally directed
towards limited concepts of efficiency and profitability might be
modified to assist the individual to be objectively and com-
passionately assessed to appreciate his qualities, and to reconcile
their significance with aspirations which may be unrealistic.

It is one of the facts of business life that the higher one goes in
an organisation, the more one is likely to be judged by the sort of
impression one creates in a particular situation rather than by the
hard facts of performance and achievement. The amount of effort
that goes into making sure there are no snags over the visit of a
more senior executive is considerable : in the environment of a
meeting, or a presentation, there is great effort to avoid bad im-
pressions about matters peripheral to the objectives of the
operation. Events like these are sources of additional tension,
which may be "normal" in the sense of being everyday, but which
may be quite irrelevant to the job being done.

In varying degrees, most companies have their methods of
jostling for position in the organisation, and sometimes managers
find it a particular burden that they are constantly having to
play office politics in order to get the ear of the boss, to get their
way with a colleague, or to resist the expansive ambitions of other
colleagues. This is particularly so in the case of technical experts
who are frequently perceived to be a threat to the status of a line
manager, rather than a resource to help him.

All the foregoing must strike a familiar chord in any manager.
But anyone who recognises the following paragraphs is causing,

or is affected by, unnecessary stress in his colleagues or in himself :

It is clear that when a man starts a new job, particularly in a new company, he is exposed to tensions of an abnormally high order, basically because he does not have the established position and well-tried routine to protect him from everyday problems. It must be nonsense that in so many companies, a manager new to the company will receive less vacation in his first year than subsequently. It can be argued that he needs more vacation in the first year in a new company than at any other time, if only to be "drawn out of the line" and given time to regroup his thoughts. When there are sudden and unexpected changes in the demands made upon an individual already established in a company, in the direction in which he is working, in the personalities with whom he has to work, and in his job responsibilities, he is subjected to an additional burden which can cause excessive pressure on him. Adaptation is not helped by the almost routine assumption that he knows how to do the new job, without instruction or help.

Some degree of personality conflict is a normal part of business life, but it is when these reach a degree of irritation and frustration that they become burdensome. This can be associated with personal failure in a particular situation resulting in criticism. It is very difficult for the person being criticised to distinguish between objective comment and personal attack, particularly if the comment, which may be justified, is expressed in an emotionally charged situation.

Conflict can result from the failure of others, perhaps on whom one has depended. It can arise in circumstances in which an individual feels he has suffered an injustice whether real or imaginary : and perhaps most painfully, it can arise in circumstances in which an individual feels his dignity has been damaged by the conduct or words of another. For some people, personality conflicts are the most painful pressures they are expected to absorb.

Fear is still a real source of anxiety to managers. In particular, the fear of obsolescence is a relatively new but very potent force. A manager may feel that he is being left behind by events; that he is not being trained to keep up with rising standards of performance; that younger and brighter people are coming in and moving ahead faster than he can hope to do. Add to these fears of redundancy. When a man gets past a certain age, he fears that his job may disappear because he is failing to perform to some new standards, because the company is uncompetitive as the result of poor management, or because a take-over may occur and he may be considered expendable.

The length of time it takes a middle aged man made redundant to obtain another acceptable position is lengthening. In 1970 it was said that it took a man of over 45 one month, for every £1,000 of salary he expected, to find a new job. That period is likely to be longer today when even men with high technical qualifications and experience are not immune. The more senior and older the man, the longer he is likely to spend job hunting.

Often there may be fears of being made a scapegoat in some crisis in the company, and fears of failure in health, which may cause a man to be unable to cope with his position. Note that this is not just a personal problem. It is likely to reduce the effectiveness of that manager in his performance. Many companies may pride themselves that they shield people from uncertainty, and that when they do have to declare a man redundant at least they have done so with a "neat stroke" which did not cause prior apprehension in the "victim". It is surprising how blind management of that style is to the fact that when it acts once in that way, everybody's security has been shaken, and remains threatened.

It may be a restatement of points already made, but it does seem to be worth emphasising that the manager who begins to recognise that he is not coping with the tasks in his job, is a man who is subject to all these abnormal tensions and begins to lose confidence and indeed to lose his way.

Individuals who make a mess of their own personal financial affairs and who have personal financial worries as a consequence, are exposed to a particularly stressful burden which often lies behind mental health problems. It is said that a man who cannot manage his own affairs, by his failure exposes probable incompetence in his job. While this may to some extent be true, the knowledge that his failure will be thus judged effectively stifles

any attempt the man might make to seek help at an early stage—
so that paradoxically his employer unknowingly steers him into
worse trouble than might otherwise be the case, if help was known
to be available without risk of censure and automatic con-
demnation. Similar remarks can be made about domestic difficulties coming on top of those already listed. It is surely the
pattern of the job that sometimes exposes the man or woman to
risks of infidelity, which would not be a temptation if family life
were less disturbed. The wife's ambition for herself may be the
cause of trouble, in that she may feel that her husband's status
demands recognition that is not forthcoming. "If X's wife has a
mink coat, why can't I?"

As the last item in this recital of abnormal stressors, consider the
sense of being trapped, dependent upon income, with a position to
maintain and with no escape from pressing on. Coping with a job
that may have become a burden; trying to keep up with colleagues when clearly not able to do so. This is often the "final
straw", particularly where other pressures have built up before
this one.

This chapter reads as a fairly gloomy catalogue, but it may promote sensitive consideration and understanding of these problems
and of the physical and mental health problems that can stem
from them. It would be appropriate perhaps to refer again to
"Peter's Principle" (defined in Chapter 4). A company with
that career planning philosophy has an inability to make an
accurate judgement of a man. The man himself has no aid or
training in assessment until he has reached a point where he
cannot cope, and then the only solution is to be taken out of the
job. In many instances this means he has to leave the company
because there is no socially acceptable pattern for allowing him
to step down to a lower job. In other companies, however, the
practice of demotion has become more acceptable. How much
more satisfactory it could be if this whole unhappy process, so
very damaging to the dignity of the individual—and, by implication, a judgement upon the company's competence—could be
avoided by a more accurate assessment of an individual's capacity.

Managers in the difficulties of the kind indicated above, may
suffer physical problems of psychosomatic origin; in other cases

there are mental health problems of many different kinds emerging. There are, however, actions that sensitive and intelligent management can take to stop reactions before they get out of control.

The most obvious precaution may be to have a medical officer who is interested and trained in problems of this kind where he can be of immediate assistance when an individual shows need of help. The value of a sensitive medical officer in the company in these circumstances is threefold : (1) he can be of immediate and direct assistance to the individual as a medical practitioner who understands the environment and the problems of that individual; (2) he can communicate expertly to other doctors who will be treating this man as their patient so that there is no danger of the doctor concerned misunderstanding the environment; (3) the medical officer in the company can explain to senior managers the significance to the organisation of events that overtook the individual.

This latter action can be taken without any departure from medical ethical codes, though it may be extremely difficult. Perhaps the greatest obstacle that such a doctor has to overcome is the lapse of time so often necessary to shield the "victim" from ready identification. Reaction to present circumstances must often be ruled out, to be stored for use in the future.

Thus the situation can be prevented or put right, and help given to create an environment in which mental stress is seen to be a "normal" occupational hazard and not something that puts a mark on a man which is ineradicable. In too many cases a man who has had a nervous breakdown at some stage in his career is a marked man who "must be watched" never to be promoted again. Such a conclusion is hardly consistent with mature and contemporary attitudes to mental health.

6

Union Attitudes

TRADES unions in the United Kingdom appreciate very highly the importance of mental health, though they would seldom express it in those terms. The whole object of trades unionism is to create an industrial climate where social justice, as a foundation of mental health, is accepted.

This position was not achieved without a struggle, and much trades union tradition is enshrined in a folk memory which (like elephants' and Irishmen's) is very long. There are scars still visible in the present attitudes of trades unions, just as the scars left by the Industrial Revolution which caused them are still visible on the face of the Land.

In their day to day work, trades unions are concerned with representing the interests of their members at factory level by means of shop stewards, at local level through union branches and trades councils, at industry level through joint industrial councils and national federations and at regional and national levels through Regional Advisory committees and the Trades Union Congress.

This representation is in itself a contribution to mental health. There is a considerable risk, as outlined in many of the essays in Ronald Fraser's "Work"[7] of workers coming to regard themselves as victims of circumstance, as slaves of the system. The fact that they are represented, that someone is fighting their battles against the system, is in itself therapeutic. The fact that they can get together within the factory or in their local branches and express themselves about management and its methods is a valuable release of tension. It is not always successful. No human activity ever is. But the wonder is not that it fails occasionally (and makes news when it does) but that it is so often successful.

While the trades unions are fully aware of the impact of changing technology on increased leisure and wage packets, they are not so acutely aware of the specific effect on mental health. The difficulty is that while noise, radiations, dust, fumes, and gas can be measured by occupational hygiene techniques, methods to study quantitatively the emotional environment have not been developed. It is only in the last ten years that knowledge of hygiene methods has become part of the stock in trade of trades unions and even in this respect they still have a long way to go. Physical and chemical standards are rising rapidly but acceptance of preventive aspects of mental health will take a lot longer because the concepts are more recent and the administrative and executive machinery to deal with them does not yet exist.

In this sombre picture, however, there are several rays of light. The first is that at the 101st annual Trades Union Congress the Chairman said :

"Where work gives little or no satisfaction to the worker, where there is no freedom to exercise talent or skill, where men and women do not determine how they do their work, where they have become merely components in the production system, they have during their working lives lost their identity as individuals. This they feel, and underlying many strikes is a protest against this unnatural environment.

"If the society in which they live does not provide them with compensation for this loss of identity, there were social consequences as well. And until we have an occupational health service committed to a study in depth of the psychological consequences of modern production methods, unrest will continue. Indeed, in the absence of these remedies, strikes are likely to continue in the process of mental and physical re-adjustment.

"Nobody who has not experienced the effects of years of confinement within the walls of mass production, without apparent means of escape, can understand the debilitating effects on the mind, the vocabulary, on the spiritual capacity of human endurance. Nobody, without this experience, can really understand why men down tools, when on the surface there seems to be only a pretext, to escape momentarily from the monotony of an unnatural existence."

This expression of the importance of psycho-social factors in the environment is further endorsed by practical measures, one of which was the establishment of the T.U.C. Institute of Occupational Health within the London School of Hygiene and Tropical Medicine, which is itself a post-graduate department of London University.

The policy of the T.U.C. is to press for the establishment of a comprehensive national occupational health service, to maintain the two-way relationship between work and health. The main difficulty in achieving this objective in this country is the fragmentation of responsibility between different government departments, so that factory legislation concerning employees is under the agency of either the Department of Employment, the Ministry of Agriculture, Food and Fisheries or the Ministry of Power, while responsibility for health is carried by the National Health Service which is part of the Department of Health and Social Security.

Trades unions are accustomed to dealing with the Department of Employment, which is the department most concerned with tripartite discussions on industrial policies. They are not accustomed to dealing with the Department of Health because they tend to regard medicine as a field of activity in which they can play no active part or make valid criticisms. A great deal of work remains to be done to change attitudes in this respect and to exercise a critical voice in the strategy of the use of medical manpower, and to understand the significance of the contribution which could be made now by the medical profession to the health of the community as a whole, or its constituent parts.

Finally, as a means of increasing understanding, the trades unions have an effective educational programme through the T.U.C. Training College, summer schools, week-end schools and through similar activities organised within individual unions. No one would pretend that this is enough. The effort has to be considerably enlarged. But enough is being done to point the way.

There are several examples of attitudes which may be out of place today. One is the suspicion of doctors in industry as agents of the employer. Another already mentioned is the perception of "Managers" as if they own the factory, or as if they were mere lackeys of the employer. Perhaps the increasing unionisation of management and clerical grades will help to convey the message that managers are workers too.

Is it not remarkable that the most stringent demand for medical certificates comes from union sick clubs? By demanding short term certificates for periods of less than three days, either employer or union obscures understanding of the withdrawal from work of an individual, who may not be "totally incapacitated" by any objective measure, but who really does not feel well enough to work.

A complication of relationships in industry is the competition between unions for membership, or within a union for representation, or endorsement as a representative. These problems have already been shown to occur in any organisation which is becoming institutionalised, and should not immediately earn the label of "anarchy".

Industry is arbitrarily defined into management and workers, and this "simple" separation is a confusing background to the study of stress at work. Obviously managers work too. They rarely have a stake in the company for which they work, so that the image of a 19th century boss applied to a 20th century manager is not appropriate. Misrepresentation and illusion exist on both sides of the division. Managers can often be rightly accused of assuming that those for whom they have a responsibility are not only subordinates, but inferiors: each "side" assumes that those on the other function in entirely different ways. But concern for money is common to both, the effect of frustration is felt by both, and each makes mistaken demands of the other. "All the firm is interested in is money" says the union negotiator, as he presses his case for a shorter working week. He often does so, not to increase time for leisure, but to create opportunities for more overtime at higher rates. His appreciation of hygiene factors and motivators is as erroneous as that of anyone else.

Differences in relationships do exist. Large numbers of manual workers report to a single manager, while the further one goes from production or simple clerical work, the fewer subordinates report to a superior, and the more complex becomes the relation between immediate colleagues. The relative importance of the factors listed also changes, but it is the sense of security which is in the foreground of the "working man's" concern.

The security of the job itself is of prime importance. The increased unemployment, and the decrease in unskilled jobs, to say nothing of the large number of jobs made obsolete by improved technology, provide an environment to which those who seek work are very sensitive. They seek work in the sense that they are not themselves able to provide the materials and processes with which they earn a living, and to that extent have no control over their future.

The period from 1945 to 1960 was a time of full employment in most parts of the United Kingdom. A greater sense of security existed, and people could believe that they had employment for the rest of their working lives. Recently, however, productivity deals, rationalisation, mergers of companies and increases of shift working are bringing back feelings of insecurity—partly because the changes tend to take place rapidly and without warning, allowing very little time to absorb and adjust to new conditions. Very little choice is left whether to accept or not.

Productivity deals tend to alter individual or group identity, which has often been obscured by viewing hourly-paid employees as soulless cyphers. Being sensitive because of the environment described, attempts to alter even simple or apparently trivial things cause bitter resistance to both management and union proposals, which may not be considered to have taken into account the proper interests of those affected by change. Conflict may arise within a union because one group is seen as "absorbing" another.

In a famous productivity agreement published in 1960,[8] one proposal was that a number of small groups of workers should be merged into a larger one in which each person would be able to do the jobs of all the others. Tube cleaners, tank cleaners, timbermen, craftsman's mates, and labourers were all to be called cleaner/labourers. Those concerned almost went on strike in response to that proposed description, but the matter appeared to be settled by renaming them as maintenance operators. Ten years later, supervisors tend to select members of the group for particular jobs on the basis of their former skill and expertise, and the men themselves think of, and refer to each other as "ex tube cleaner" or "ex timberman", so perpetuating their "old" identity.

When the job content is changed other anxieties are caused. Younger people faced with a new job doubt their ability to do it, and this fear of a new technique is much greater in the older man, who has become set for many years in one familiar routine, and who has doubts about his ability to learn. While younger workers are both more resilient and accustomed to change, there may be fear that "before I've learned this job, they'll change it again". The choice of suitable jobs available decreases as one becomes older, so that paradoxically those most likely to be affected by obsolescence are those with least opportunity to look after themselves by being able to choose from a wide range of alternatives.

Shift work of varying cycles[9] also tends to increase as expensive machinery requires 24-hour operation to be economical. An Australian worker summed up the type of feelings common among shift workers in the following manner:

"As a shift worker my world is an endless round of changing shifts in which family and personal life suffer most. The confusion of weekly changing shifts, sleeping and eating habits, is further heightened by the often unfilled demands of a growing family. I have largely had to forego the companionship of my sons while they are young, so that they now look outside the home for many of the things that I would like to give them. My wife, who has had to work during most of our married life, has also missed many of the social contacts which are necessary for a happy life.

"Unfortunately, the result has been that our family life has degenerated into an unreal existence of club life for my wife and myself and a street corner existence for my sons. The hopeless part of it all is that I have no particular skill and have to work shifts to maintain my present earnings. Although I would like to find straight day work I just couldn't afford to take the resultant loss in earnings. Another thing that bothers me is the thought that most of my fellow workers and myself are just "getting by" although we are living in a booming economy. If this is prosperity, I wonder what would happen if the economy should level off or decline?"

It is easy to dismiss this problem by assuming that the answer is for such a man to give up shift work. Even if there is day work conveniently available, the increased earnings to be gained from shiftwork, piecework, and overtime set the standard of living which generally exceeds that possible on basic rates. To some extent, dependance on these extras adds further reasons for conflict, since overtime is likely to be associated with high demand for production, and is the first reduction to be made by management to cope with falling sales. It would be bad enough if this were the only variable acting on overtime but its allocation to individuals or groups, by management or unions, causes jealousies, and withholding overtime is often used by either union or management as a punishment or sanction.

In many industrial negotiations safety measures for the employees have a low priority, but it does not follow that good working conditions breed a good relationship between worker and management, or that bad working conditions are a symptom of bad relations between the two parties.

At a firm of vehicle builders with about 240 employees, the working conditions were appalling, but the workers and the management were on good terms—perhaps because in a small company the boss knew all his workers, and visited them every day and chatted with them. Here is an extract from a study group's report on this firm's working conditions :

"Immediately on entering the works, unsafe working practices cried out for attention. Welders sparked happily behind non-existent flash screens, content in the hope that fires started by their sparks would be quickly put out by an impressive array of empty extinguishers on the wall !

Men operated a dozen grinding wheels without goggles, though they were available.

Ventilation in the vehicle spray shop depended on the vagaries of the winds. When the westerly blew, overspray from the paint shop carried through into the main workshop, often damaging finished vehicles.

Despite their lack of protection, sand shoes were the order of the day—worn no doubt to allow the workers to leap over areas overcrowded with raw materials. Workers enjoyed their sandwiches relaxed over the work bench rather than use the lunch room. Nobody bothered to wash their hands, probably from fear of catching some disease from the unsanitary washroom.

Calls of nature certainly didn't waste much productive working time—the stench from the outhouses was nauseating. These units stood, understandably, in great isolation in the backyard. It is inconceivable that this factory has been examined recently by competent factory inspectors. Yet, despite the dozen or more hazards that were located in the visit, the employees and the unions tolerate these conditions, secure in the knowledge that when the inevitable accident occurs, the State will care for them."

In contrast to this example, at another factory where conditions were almost clinical, the same working party found the work force to be unhappy. Several explanations were suggested. A period of redundancy and rationalisation had just occurred, and management became more distant from the worker in the re-organisation. The modern plant did not compensate for the deterioration in personal relationships, which were made even worse by the isolation from fellow workers caused by automated machinery, either by distance, or the interference with human conversation caused by the chatter of the machines.

In an earlier chapter, the texture of the environment, the web of the structure of the organisation, and the difficulties of communication have been described. Such problems affect not only the big companies, but groups of workers themselves as they grow bigger. Unions and industries are becoming bigger institutions, and have not yet learnt to communicate properly either with their members or employees. Both may come to decisions about individuals in their organisation without taking into account their real interests, either because opinions are not sought, or because views are misrepresented or misunderstood.

Uncertainty, apathy, fear and insolence are common in situations such as the "unofficial" strikes by dockers, who may feel that their officials are not expressing the views of the membership, nor their concern that their livelihoods were threatened by alterations in jobs due to containerisation. Attention to these problems must take the identity of the worker, and his role, into consideration. One man can be at different times a member of the public, or of a union, or of a church, or a husband, or a voter, and so on. One union may affect a public made up of members of other unions, but industrial disputes tend to be viewed as if only one role were valid.

The social system has elsewhere been shown to be dynamic, and until argument and agreement are based upon change as a fundamental feature of life, rigid structures will be cracked or broken. By "freezing" a man into one brittle role today, he becomes liable to fragment into a social problem tomorrow. Just as his roles change or overlap, so do jobs, so that instead of the former "my job was my life" custom, the worker may in future successfully engage in several different jobs during his lifetime.

7

Identity and Status

THE objective of this chapter is to hint at influences upon people as they work together, or engage in conflict.

An individual plays many roles throughout his life. Some are confined to particular age groups, others are determined by chance, others again are chosen. These many roles summate together to form a complete person, and are conveyed by him to those around him, so that the role he is in at any time is signalled by speech, appearance, behaviour, or dress. The sergeant major shouts commands which are evidently to be obeyed; the infantryman wearing a bearskin hat in days gone by did so to appear taller, and so more frightening, to his opponent; the wigs and gowns of judge and counsel in court express the solemnity and importance of that institution; and "respect for the cloth" recognises a man's special relationship between God and other men.

At any time then, a person may signal a role that he currently plays, but whatever that signal may be, it may be misinterpreted. The hippie might perceive the sergeant major as merely a noise threat to the environment, uniforms and robes may no longer be held in awe, and clerical dress may seem an anachronistic irrelevance. Furthermore, a role which is not being signalled may be assumed by those who are mistaken by perceiving signals incorrectly. Have you ever thought you saw a clergyman in the street only to find that the passerby was wearing dark clothes with no tie? Are you ever surprised when you see young men in suits, collars and ties emerging from factories which used to disgorge men in cloth caps and overalls? Would you be upset if a doctor visited you by appointment wearing dirty overalls?

In organisations, these signals become more formalised. Old school ties, membership of clubs, presence of a carpet in a civil servant's office, the type of car driven, the bowler hat and umbrella, all these things convey an individual role and status and in some cases imply that others have endorsed the claim.

More subtle than these manifestations of group identity or status are those which exist or may be thought to be distinguished by more subtle marks. Whatever the accent, there are U and non-U expressions. Membership of an aristocratic family may not appear to be compatible with egalitarian philosophy to the observer whose own convictions cloud his judgement. Most important of all in industry is the assumption by "workers" that their fellow promoted to foreman has changed sides, or indeed the converse assumption by his manager that he has not yet abandoned old prejudices quickly enough or that he is still "too familiar" with the men. In earlier days this alteration of role would have been expressed by the purchase of a bowler to replace a cloth cap.

Situations such as this exemplify many in which a "reference group" determines to some extent the expected behaviour of the individual who belongs, or has belonged, to it. Ex-public schoolboys, men who have served in the armed forces, men who have given colonial service, all are expected by their fellows to behave in a particular way, to conform to various rules, to hold similar ethical values. This expectation exerts a subtle pressure which helps the individual to live up to those expectations, "to do what has to be done", or "not to let the side down".

Others witnessing a particular behaviour pattern will conclude that many things associated in fact or fiction with that behaviour pattern are true whatever the evidence to the contrary. "The Irish sleep with the pigs." "Coloured people are dirty." "Employers only understand one thing—money." "High Court judges don't understand workers because they've never done a day's work." The list of possible false assumptions is endless, and the effective barrier set up between people who do not question those assumptions can disrupt any attempts at understanding, and can provoke or prolong conflict unnecessarily.

Membership of a group is gained by self-selection, or selection by others. Interview before employment, sponsoring for membership of a club, examination for entry to a profession, all are selection procedures. Those who decide to live in a particular suburb, or are regular customers of a particular public house, set up or join a group themselves, and having done so, may set up unspoken selection procedures to maintain cohesion. Of course, active and passive selection both operate together, as for instance in applying for a job. The applicant chooses the job, and is then chosen, from among others. The criteria of choice reflect the objectives of the organisation, and in some instances are intended to select not only intellectual qualifications, but those of personality, and indeed the spouse's personality as well.

Psychological assessment systems are numerous, and some even sensational! They range from aptitude tests and intelligence tests, to personality inventories of a most complex nature, which assess several hundred characteristics and compute the results into defined categories. Sometimes several elements are combined, so that a group exercise suggests the "best" member of that group for the job to be done.

In certain of the management courses described later on, such groups or syndicates undertake tasks, and both the process and content of the resulting group interaction may be commented upon by a trained observer. Such an exercise is the basis for Phase I of the Blake Managerial Grid (described more fully in Chapter 10). The description of another example of such an exercise may illustrate many of the influences working upon individuals undertaking what appeared to be a very simple task, which nevertheless demonstrated much that was unspoken.

The group concerned consisted of about twenty doctors attending a post-graduate course. They came from several continents, and perhaps a third were of European origin. The remainder was made up of Africans and Asians from several countries. All were men, and they were each asked to write down five features of their work which satisfied them, and to rank these in order of importance.

This was to be done individually, so that a piece of paper would record that individual's personal ranking of factors which he himself had identified. The group was then asked to split into two halves, and it was left to the class to choose how the two

groups should be composed. Two members began to collect teams
around themselves, by choosing those one or two close acquaintances that each had already made during the academic year.
Each of the two "leaders" were European, one a service officer of
fairly senior rank, and of early middle age, with substantial
experience. The other was a younger man, with some experience
in hospital and in a research institute. He often expressed what
he described as radical socialist ideas, and throughout the
academic year had frequently posed fundamental questions,
either in informal conversations, or in the course of the scholastic
curriculum.

It is important here to emphasise that what follows is a
tentative interpretation of what took place. Too often, the commentator appears to present the one valid interpretation, either
by his authority, or in the perception of those listening to him. It
is sometimes regrettable that clearer disclaimers are not specified,
because interpretation of so many variables operating at one
time is determined by the perception of the commentator, and
whatever his claim to authority, may not be the only possible
explanation.

To return to the doctors; each group was asked to discuss the
individual rankings of the five factors bestowing work satisfaction,
and to agree a group list of five, derived from the greater number
appearing in personal lists, and to agree a group assessment of
priorities. So that the two groups might work separately, one was
asked to remain in their usual classroom, while the other group
used another room.

The group which stayed in its familiar room was that led by
the younger man. The whole class throughout the year demonstrated a preference for tutorial and participative learning, so
that tables and chairs were in no particular order, (though when-
ever there was a formal lecture, Europeans gravitated to the
back!). Perhaps by chance, perhaps because of familiarity with
the usual informality of the room, this first group adopted positions approximately in a circle, and discussion was informal;
there was no obvious chairman, people spoke when they had
something to say, and if a response was made, it was directed by
the respondent directly to the person who had made the original

statement. No such member had any particular role, claimed by himself or bestowed on him by others, and discussion flowed freely.

It was possibly characteristic both of the style of the man who chose the group, and of the unstructured process of the discussion itself, that this group was ready to argue its case when the time allowed had elapsed. But this "efficiency" was easier for this particular group, who had not as yet agreed a priority list of five satisfying factors in the group's lives, which they realised operated in different ways at various times and according to circumstances.

Meanwhile the second group, led by the officer, made their way (not in step!) to the other classroom, which was set out in traditional manner, with all seats facing a large, clean blackboard. This group sent one of its members to the blackboard, where all the factors derived from personal lists were set down, and a certain amount of classification resulted from interaction between individuals in the class, and the man at the blackboard. Their re-titling and ranking was not finished in the time allowed, but they had agreed the factors in the upper section of their priorities. Under some pressure from the perpetrator of the whole exercise, this group were persuaded to return to the usual classroom, where their rivals awaited them.

On re-entering the room the first group were already established in their places, and merely had to reorientate the chairs towards the next part of the exercise. Those returning, though they scattered to various part of the room, did not disrupt the cohesion, however informal, of those already there; but neither could it maintain the relationship in space between its members established in the borrowed classroom. Each group had been asked to nominate a single representative to argue each group's list of priorities with a view to establishing a ranking of factors agreed by the total class, and both groups had chosen, or had acknowledged, their leader for the task.

Each representative was now expected to express his group's views, and to win or to yield various points in arriving at a conclusion. The cohesion of the members of one block, close to their nominee, and the disintegration and scattering of the second group, some of whom were separated from their representative by

members of the opposition, might have had some effect in this
instance, but it is only possible to speculate. However, the disadvantage any delegation might suffer, on being invited to join
another delegation already established in a room, might in other
cases be a significant factor in the process of debate.

In the case under consideration each was to be the sole speaker
on his group's behalf, and his constituency were to observe how
the debate went, but were forbidden to participate themselves.
Thus it was hoped they would have an opportunity to learn
something of the forces at work when representatives meet, and
they would also have a potent effect upon those representatives.
The latter might remember or forget points considered by one
or more of his constituency to be important. They were not only
supporting him, they were anxious that he should support them.
He would be in a similar position, trying to represent the views
of others with as much sincerity as his own, while yet being fearful
that his constituents might not perceive his performance as being
either fair or adequate.

The positions the two adversaries took up was itself interesting.
The officer sat in the place he had usually occupied throughout
the academic year. The other man sat casually on the end of the
table, which usually served as a desk for his opponent (shared
with another service officer!). In that position the "casual" man
on the table, literally spoke down from on high, to a man who was
his senior in age and experience, who was correctly seated for
serious discussion.

To some extent the debate which followed was artificial, in
that both were aware that they were being watched, and that
their conversation was only an exercise. Attitude to the task
undertaken is an important factor in any team exercise, or
negotiation. Examples include race, religion and political conviction; status and rank within the group to which one predominantly belongs; nationality, cultural background, social
class all have their effect, derived from or reinforced by past
experience and education, which is even further distinguished by
school or university. It was remarkable that when the exercise
here described had been proposed to the whole class, at the beginning of the day, and without previous warning, they had

varied widely (and obviously) in their interest. Some may have
felt that the use of a whole morning for such activity was an
impediment to passing the forthcoming examination in other
subjects. Others no doubt suspected the competence of the man
who had engineered the thing, since the whole class had already
reason to doubt the relevance of psychology and all its pomps!

However, the two adversaries duly debated their priorities, only
the first two of which need be discussed here. The "formal"
group ranked the satisfaction of the practice of medicine itself
after the salary and standard of living enjoyed by doctors. In a
burst of generous frankness, their leader confessed that at first
salary had ranked first, but that in private his group had decided
that they would appear mercenary, lesser, men if they were to
express such avarice. But the significance of that jocose remark
should not be underestimated, for the group had demonstrated
spontaneously that whatever their conviction, there was an
expectation by others that they should behave otherwise.

The "informal" group leader took an unexpected stance. His
group had recognised different rankings depending upon circumstances, and he now debated not the ranking, but the neces-
sity or relevance to rank at all! Negotiation thus progressed
without conclusion, not that there was deadlock, but because
there was no hope of reconciliation of the different views. But one
immortal moment of dialogue remains. One stated " 'X' follows
logically from 'Y'." "Ah yes," replied his courteous opponent
"*But* ... !"

Before leaving the subject of roles and groups, it may be of
value to make a few general remarks concerning influences on
group behaviour perhaps only suggested in recounting the experience of the twenty doctors. On an undoubtedly grander scale,
consider for a moment the difference between the two party
system of politics which led to, and is preserved by, the House of
Commons. The Government benches are occupied by the
majority party, regardless of its representation. The picturesque
and constitutional manner of debate is controlled by tradition.
Physical violence is prevented by the lines, drawn two sword's
lengths apart, woven into the carpet in front of each front bench.
Personal vilification is to some extent modified both by the

procedure of addressing remarks to the speaker, and by reference to "the Honourable Member for . . ." rather than naming the individual under attack.

The Speaker controls debate, by indicating who is to speak next, and any speech in the House is directed by one member, in the direction of those on the other side of the House who can all see him.

Contrast this with the stability of Governments who are ranged in a semicircle. While benches in the House of Commons indicate the rank of those on them, each seat of those who have adopted a semicircular debating chamber indicate not only rank, but *degree* of political conservatism or revolutionary intent. Except at the extreme wings of such a room, one cannot face opposition directly, and the boundary between that opposition and one's allies is indistinct. There is a predisposition to coalitions, which are unusual in British politics. The voting system of the House of Commons declares a man to all members as an "Aye" or a "No" or an abstainer, because the latter must remain in his seat, while the others actually leave the chamber to record their vote. Further, there is room for less than the full number of Members in the House, who sit on benches, not in chairs. Thus the House is not distractingly empty when less than full membership is present.

King Arthur had a round table, and the principle implied operates in many a conference today, in which it might otherwise be difficult to give the honour he expects, to the most important member present, because several claim to be that person. The Vietnam peace conference in Paris was delayed for weeks by debate upon the shape of the table, because one of the parties whose presence was demanded by another, was unacceptable at a round table by the third party. North Vietnam insist that they help "indigenous freedom fighters" in South Vietnam. Clearly they cannot sit mixed with them on one side of a table, "they are a force in their own right". The United States disagrees; "The Freedom Fighters are invaders from North Vietnam, obviously they must be represented by the North Vietnamese delegation itself". Such political wrangling is a product of human behaviour.

At lesser negotiations, different arrangements may be made. In persuading children to learn, one school may focus the attention of rows of pupils upon the teacher and blackboard they face. Another school attempts to focus the children's attention on tasks shared by groups around tables, which are visited from time to time by the teacher. The atmosphere, quality of learning, and discipline are clearly distinguishable on entering the room; and that statement is not intended to judge either way, for at Eton, four classes go on at one time in one room, on four subjects, facing four teachers dispersed at the four corners of the compass!

Territorial sense is more common than one appreciates. Father in some traditional households still has "his" chair. Members of Pall Mall clubs have their places in reading rooms. Even when it is not mentioned as part of a management course, the members of syndicates tend to establish individual positions. And when "management" meets "union" it is "across the negotiating table", drawn up in ranks. On occasions when a "neutral" specialist is invited to attend, each side hope that he will "join" it.

In describing some of the activity of groups, communication is obviously important, and examples have been given. Sometimes silence is interpreted as a decision by the silent one to withdraw from the group, and may provoke bitter attack, unless it has been established that the very occasional comment made by such a person is worth waiting for.

The "task oriented"[10] group depends for its effectiveness on a clear definition of its task. Leadership may rest upon one man, or may successfully rotate, to be held with the approval of others by the member who has demonstrated competence upon the particular contribution he is making at the time. Whether fixed upon a chairman, or exercised by members of the group in turn, the group's effort must remain directed towards the achievable task. Dispute is constructive and apposite, and is not allowed to degenerate into pointless or inappropriate squabbling. While the task is perceptible, and considered capable of solution, the task oriented group tends to be realistic, to be aware of the outside world, both in terms of its effect upon the group, and terms of the groups' hope to influence it in turn.

Should the group be unable to perform the task or solve the problem, or should its task be ill defined in the first place, it tends to adopt an attitude of "basic assumptions" in which the outside world becomes almost coincidental. It becomes unable to recognise the unthinkable, that its work will not have any effect, but behaves as if its deliberations will in some way be of use. It begins to turn in on itself, and so to justify its existence. It becomes more concerned with its own needs and those of its members, so that there is inappropriate expression of sympathy with members who arrive late, or have been away, or have difficulties of some sort. By so misdirecting its activity, it lessens further the likelihood of having a constructive effect upon the real world and slides down a spiral to insignificance.

One of the paths by which the "task" group deteriorates is that followed when the task exceeds the competence of the group to cope with it; an outside expert is co-opted, or the leader of the group itself is vested with a special authority, which may get out of hand to the point of depriving the members of the group of what skills they did have. By this process of "de-skilling" the authority is perceived as being the only source of the answer, and sometimes progresses even further, so that members of the group adopt an attitude of not understanding what the authority, or now even other members of the group, are saying. This may be explicitly expressed, "What are we talking about?"

One last word to chairmen. Having successfully maintained order, having channelled even the most heated debate to the matter in hand, sum up in terms of the statement "I think we have concluded that. . . ." Members of the meeting are then offered an opportunity to disagree, even if they don't take it. If, on the contrary, the chairman feels it is necessary to end a meeting he can use the phrase "We appear to have agreed that. . . ." Skilfully done, he allows members to recognise glimpses of their selected contribution as a consensus with which they cannot disagree for fear of appearing to be going back upon what they said earlier.

8

Women's Equality

EQUALITY of opportunity for the sexes is a cause which demands support, but enthusiasm must not ignore the real differences between men and women. Difference in muscular strength, physical effort capacity, manual dexterity and patience are obvious. The comparability of ageing physiology is less obvious. For the woman, the end of her childbearing capability is recognisable more easily than the less well defined involution of the ageing male, but the less dramatic climacteric he suffers nonetheless puts him at a disadvantage at what may be a critical time in his life.

Two world wars have contributed greatly to women's emancipation. Though not yet complete, it is less remarkable to see women in senior posts, or as eminent scholars, or doing some jobs assumed until recently to be the exclusive reserve of men. However it is still "news" when a Russian airliner lands in London with a woman pilot, while the American space programme has not included a flight by a woman.

A study of the effect of reproductive life upon a woman[11] suggests that for a few days before her menstrual period a woman becomes more tense, and more accident prone, while at the same time suffering some impairment of intellect, manifest in a decrease of the quality of decision. Yet again, the variation that exists between people must be emphasised, and some reserve about the findings of such surveys has been expressed by those who point out that the woman whose attention is directed to her periods may be affected by that preoccupation, rather than by her otherwise normal physiological functions themselves.

Certainly, a number of successful career women would not agree that their performance is substandard for up to one working week in four, and many ambitious women would resent very much a suggestion that their premenstrual incapacity is such that they should avoid decision making at that time. Perhaps a reasonable reconciliation of theory and practice would be for men and women both to be aware that menstruation is a phenomenon which may affect performance. For the woman concerned, perhaps awareness of the significance of her condition will make it possible for her to compensate adequately when necessary, and to control increased irritability, or to avoid where possible particular emotional strain.

Assuming then that the adolescent and reproductive woman understands the significance of her reproductive capability to the work she is doing, there are two other stages in her life which themselves merit more attention.

Woman's role in renewing the community to which she belongs is less well defined in the context of the population explosion. In some countries that role has been recognised to the extent that a pregnant woman continues to receive pay from her erstwhile employer for several months after her delivery. Elsewhere, considerable effort by the community provides care for children in Kibbutzim, or in day nurseries. These efforts certainly reduce many of the anxieties of young people who might otherwise have been unable to have children without suffering a considerable drop in their standard of living.

It will be interesting to see whether the increasing volume of propaganda to discourage reproduction will cause significant frustration in those upon whom sanctions will doubtless be brought to bear. There is already an implied accusation of antisocial behaviour; the reversal of social security benefits is being debated; and the community is thus setting objectives which are contrary to those of many people. This conflict does not help an organisation which may want to recognise woman's maternal role by providing or improving maternity benefits, whether they are financial in terms of pay or pension rights, or whether they merely postulate unbroken service and job security.

The menopause in women, and the climacteric in men, are colloquially and accurately described as the change of life. In a world dominated by males, recognition of their own physiology has been denied by men, perhaps because the parallel with "frail" woman implied unmanly weakness. Perhaps women's increasing ability to voice criticism, and certainly advances in physiological studies, have produced incontrovertible evidence that men do undergo a significant regression, though it may start later, and last longer, than the female involution.

Experience of the climacteric in both sexes varies between individuals, and affects others around them in different ways. Those working in problems of sex and marriage are no longer surprised, but still remark the degree to which communication between couples married for years is blocked by taboos or embarrassment. Whether formalised by marriage or not, relationships between adults, and between them and their children are more profound and intense than any others.

No amount of sexual emancipation will facilitate the task of putting up with someone else at close range for a prolonged period.[12] Personalities interact, and if incompatible, reject each other. Otherwise there is a constant process of adjustment, sometimes by one, sometimes by the other, as an understanding of each other's drives, ambitions, intellectual and emotional life increases. In a large number of cases, the "understanding" is reached by choosing to ignore that a difference exists. Sometimes the suppression, conscious or unconscious, can no longer be maintained while coping with other pressures. Thus it was possible that the method by which a man tackled a boiled egg at breakfast each morning for years became suddenly significant enough to be cited as evidence of cruelty in a divorce suit!

Such petty irritations are commonplace, and fortunately more often than not they are recognised as such, and accepted by the parties concerned. At the menopause, the woman's change of mood or behaviour may present her spouse with several problems to contend with at once, and it is characteristic of the woman's psychological and physiological adaptation that its various components get out of step, and each may vary erratically. Thus she really may not know what she wants; she may really react to similar situations in different ways; and her husband in trying to satisfy her whim of yesterday, finds that he is annoying her intensely, or "being unreasonable" today.

The woman who is at work at this time in her life, has to contend with the emotional adjustments while attempting to maintain consistent performance in her job. These difficulties are faced by men in their turn, but either sex, single, widowed, or separated, may receive very little help when they need it. Women supervisors run the risk of being pronounced "bitches" by those in their care, who may themselves one day suffer the same fate; secretaries may be criticised by the boss for becoming too emotional; men will be judged to have become crotchety in their old age.

Few indeed will be those who recognise their subordinate in the role of a spouse contending with the mid-life crisis in his partner. Earlier in this book the inappropriateness of the concept of "industrial" stress has been mentioned. Those who go out to work are complete personalities. They do not change on crossing the threshold of the office, or when clocking in or out at the factory gate. A row at home may change behaviour at work, and a "bad day at the office" or a "lousy job that had to be done" have their effect on behaviour at home.

All this may seem obvious. No new statement has been made, and yet there is a need for greater understanding which is so obviously lacking. How many managers authorising sick pay, or contending with absenteeism, consciously bear in mind the difficulties an older woman may have in contending with irregular, and perhaps suddenly copious periods? How many attempt to understand or even recognise emotional strain imposed by that risk?

In Yugoslavia, women's associations do not have to fight for the right to vote, or for equal pay, or for equality in law of children born in or out of wedlock. All these, and free abortion, were provided by law immediately after the second world war. Nevertheless, they do have to press for implementation of laws already made, and for various services to assist women who work, or for institutions to care for their children. It was improvement of the position, rather than establishment of new attitudes, which was the aim of one women's association.

That association was able to demonstrate that despite the favourable laws, larger factories avoided employing women, particularly if they had large families. Pregnant women were even less welcome, because health and social needs predisposed to absenteeism. Some of the services which should have been provided by firms were not made available on economic grounds. Only a few women were elected to workers' councils, and even fewer had the benefits of technical training enjoyed by equivalent male workers. In the hope that a meeting of management sponsored by the association might lead to greater understanding, a series of papers on the various problems was commissioned. These papers did not materialise, because it was evident that management knew the problems already, and that it was understanding, not facts, that was required at work or at home. This lack of conviction, so unsatisfactory to the women concerned, might be perpetuated indefinitely, since those who made decisions were managers, and the vast majority of managers were men.

The association reconsidered their proposal, and posed several questions some months later. If understanding was the problem, how might it be promoted? When women work so often to provide the "extras" which determine their families' standard of living, why do they have such difficulty in being involved in decisions which affect them? With these new questions before them, managers did meet the women's association for discussion which was at first very difficult. After all, if the problem was lack of understanding, how could comprehension be gained?

The slow start led to complex debate, which need only be summarised here. Basically it seemed that there was a fear of change. Over thousands of years, men's attitude to women was one of superiority. The emotional and instinctive roots of this prejudice are deeply ingrained, to the extent that recognition and commitment to equality would not be recognised as an actual enhancement of women's position, but would be perceived as a threat of the men's diminution. Resulting attitudes were not to be changed by a stroke of the legislative pen. Nor were socio-political beliefs sufficient to change the attitude. Immediately after the war, man had agreed the equality of women, but this was done at an intellectual level. It had seemed logical at the time that "no one can be allowed to subject, exploit, or underestimate anyone else", and no doubt that included women. At a political

level, men had preached equality for a quarter of a century, but
previous centuries had convinced men that women were inferior,
and had led them to take women for granted, and so underestimate their contribution.

The process of the debate just described is also of interest. As
might have been expected, almost all those in the discussion were
able to demonstrate prejudice by several examples. Emotions
were roused, and one woman who had "betrayed" the women's
group by a contentious statement, was herself accused of having
anti-feminist prejudice. Tempers flared, and as so often is the
case, an objective opinion was interpreted as a personal attack.
The realisation that there were divisions within the two parties
confronting each other only served to raise the temperature, and
to provoke very emotional outbursts. Fortunately a coffee break
served as an interval in which tempers cooled, and later those
concerned were able to recognise and appreciate that many of the
arguments expressed on both sides had themselves been rigid,
conservative, or even hypocritical. In one instance one woman
became aware that her own attitudes to unmarried mothers had
been to some extent determined by her schoolteacher who, thrice
married yet childless, condemned the provision of care for unmarried mothers.

Having demonstrated for themselves how attitudes may be
formed in childhood and developed in adolescence, those at the
discussion were able to consider how such ingrained attitudes
might be changed. It became evident that change was a long
process, the rate of which might be increased if the right approach
were chosen.

Moreover, the shorter the term of the prejudice, the more
amenable to change it might be. If followed that hope rested with
the younger generation who were accustomed by the concept of
equality, and that the appointment of younger managers might
serve to hasten change. But even that is only a beginning, since
individuals remain with personal and perhaps internal conflicts
to resolve. One example quoted referred to one of the towns
devastated in recent earthquakes. An appeal was launched to
rebuild the maternity hospital which had been totally destroyed.
No one disagreed that this was a good cause, and no one ques-

tioned the maternal basis of female physiology. Yet older people were heard to say to the fund collector, "let me give you my subscription later, when no one can see me", or "here's my subscription, but don't add my name to the list". One possible explanation for this unwillingness to be seen to contribute was that such older workers were affected by their own inability to conceive.

Finally, the meeting considered the part the women themselves should play in changing attitudes. Women are not educated to participate in society, but receive an education said to be appropriate for girls as distinct from boys. Men and women would have to learn to see as part of their task, efforts to improve their own position in the community.

In arriving at these conclusions, those participating in the meeting had learned much. The women's association members realised that their work was no longer merely to report, inform, and persuade. The challenge was far greater, and new problems had only begun.

9

Communication

TO some extent appreciation of the importance of communication between people is distorted by the frequent occurrence of the word as current jargon. Those liberals and radicals who use the word frequently in conversation and interview, and who profess to be trying to "communicate", seem often to fail to enlighten those to whom they speak about the meaning and purpose of their life style.

At the simplest level, conversation in plain language can be misunderstood. The physical properties of sound are demonstrated in whispering galleries in which the voice carries for long distances preserved by the properties of the space through which it travels. The distortion of sound may lead to misunderstanding of the message. An Army signal "Send reinforcements, I'm going to advance" is said to have been interpreted as "Send three and fourpence, I'm going to a dance." Superimposed upon the physical distortion of the sound waves themselves is the expectation in the listener's mind of what he is about to hear.

All sorts of unspoken signs accompany conversation, so that one would not expect the statement "I love you" to come from a face contorted with rage. The movements of the mouth may be fundamental to the lip reading practiced by the deaf, but it plays a part in conversation among those who can hear as well. Frequently in a room crowded with people in animated conversation, one catches a glimpse of the face of someone at a distance, whose words become more distinct in what was before an unintelligible babble of background noise.

It is also possible to demonstrate that in one's own language, one can interpret conversation from separate syllables with blanks in between, because familiar cadenzas of speech are heard in a sort of audible shorthand. Indeed, despite Victor Borge's attempts to provide them, there is no need in speech for punctuation marks, which are conveyed instead by inflection and tempo. The conversion of conversation, or a prepared speech, into written prose is a task which has caused stress in at least one author!

Language may be a further complication. Interpretors are familiar with the pitfall represented by a word which is almost identical in two languages, but which conveys a totally different message to each of those conversing. An example is the word "anthropology". In Anglo-Saxon minds, the word refers to a study of man, his development, his way of life and social history. To a Frenchman, l'anthropologie equates with the Anglo-Saxon word anthropometry, the study of the dimensions and growth of the body of the human animal.

Oratory, particularly when it has political aims, is notorious for the way in which a simple statement of fact can be so loaded with emotion by the way in which it is expressed, or the circumstances in which it is made. "Christ was a Jew" is a simple historical fact which few would bother to dispute, and which might therefore be considered something not meriting mention. Yet in the 1930s in the East End of London, those same four words became an emotional slogan to counter anti-semitic activities in that area. More recently the term "affluent society" is sometimes interpreted cynically or with derision to direct attention to a part of society which cannot be so described.

The community made up of so many sub-groups and individuals as a nation has a common language only in a limited sense. Not everyone has access to, or respect for, definitions of words which appear in dictionaries. "Workers" defined theoretically in a dictionary are subdivided in practice into those who consider themselves to be workers in the sense of physical labour. Those who work all day in offices, or shopkeepers, or dentists, or architects, are excluded by those who claim the exclusive title; and by doing so, an obstruction is put in the way of free communication between all those who really do work in the dictionary sense. This obstacle is one of perception, since the so called "worker" would concede the dictionary definition if it was the semantics which became the subject of debate.

The language, common in that limited sense to the inhabitants of a country, reflects a culture from which it has grown, and by becoming an institute with rules of grammar and syntax, tends to perpetuate the culture that begat it.

This problem was well demonstrated in a sensitivity training laboratory set up to study problems posed by mixing people of different nationalities in management teams. Elsewhere the "T group" process is described more fully; sufficient here to report that interpersonal tensions tend to grow to a crescendo on about the third day, when a sort of crisis of criticism occurs, inhibition to expression is reduced, and an atmosphere of frank discussion is established.

At least two differences between European and Anglo-Saxon participants were experienced at one particular laboratory, and these differences can be traced to cultural differences between the continent of Europe on the one hand and the Atlantic Community, which includes Britain, on the other.

Participants were expected to wear nameplates, so that one could recognise "Jim", "Bill" and "Mac". The composition of such informal titles came more easily to the Atlantic citizens than to those of mainland Europe, one of whose nameplates contained his full title and professional address. In an interesting series of articles a French author[13] has drawn attention to the differences in philosophy between the two ethnological groups here described. He points out that in a scientific paper, a continental European will stick strictly to the point at an intellectual level throughout, while the Anglo-Saxon will not consider it odd to include the light relief of anecdote or joke. Such humour is dignified with special importance by Blake and Moulton in the Managerial Grid system of management training referred to elsewhere. These authors consider it as one of six basic factors which determine management style.

The experience of the multi-national "T" group seemed to support this hypothesis, for humorous comment could sometimes express criticism which might otherwise be more painful. The continental luminary mentioned above, whose nameplate resembled more a tombstone, introduced himself in conversation "I am a professor, but please don't call me Professor." On the second day of the course an Anglo-Saxon said "I am not a professor, but please call me 'Professor'." The gentleman concerned was just as amused by this outburst as everyone else, and learned that the formality of his background, education, and status represented a barrier to free communication between himself and others. His formal claim to status was by no means personal pomposity, but was to a great extent determined by his nationality and language. A national group in the laboratory suffered the same experience. While Anglo-Saxons on the third day were accusing each other of talking too much, of bullying, of being arrogant bastards, the European national group were still debating whether to address each other without the prefix Mr., Doctor or Professor, and were not yet able to exchange views on more important topics.

Difficulties of communication between strangers from different backgrounds experienced at the Windsor seminar were further complicated in one small discussion group by the presence of five nationalities. This mixed group was asked to consider problems of communication, and their experience is of interest. They noted that they had already become acquainted before tackling the problem, and that the trust existing between them made it easier for individuals to express controversial views. They also noted that the need to talk to establish status was the less, and they drew a parallel with the interaction between superior and subordinate. If the former does not have to emphasise his status by speech, he develops the power not only to hear the sound of someone else's voice, but also to listen to what he is saying. Many were aware that "There are none so deaf as those who will not hear", but their experience at Windsor has led them to fuller understanding of that message. Another advantage was recognised in that these acquaintances were more easily able to communicate across professional demarcation lines than might their colleagues in other organisations who had not developed *in action* the links indicated in *theory* on organisational structure charts.

Contrary to this spirit of co-operation, the group was concerned for a short time as to who should sit where. This problem was resolved, but it is noteworthy that after a break for dinner, each member of the group reclaimed "his" place. That item of the agenda being disposed of, the group set out to review current systems of communication within organisations in different lands. Having done so, they hoped to draw some general conclusions upon which recommendations for the future might be based.

The Dutch experience suggested less communication between managers and the managed than between managers and various specialists on the problems of those managed. Organisation seemed to be much more structured than that in Britain, and seemed to be accepted in that form by both employer and employee. Here was just another example of the interdependence of formality of culture, and the distinctions maintained by that formal structure. It seemed that management was expected by the unions to seek specialist help, and that the status of the specialist would help the union to accept the specialist's recommendation. At first glance such a situation would seem to be entirely foreign to the British way of industrial life but it is not so. The problem of absenteeism in Britain is treated in the same way. Both employers and employed look to the doctor for an answer because "Sickness absence is his problem, not ours!" This despite the fact that short term absence attributed to sickness has been demonstrated beyond reasonable doubt to be a voluntary withdrawal from work.

So it is that in Holland steering or task committees of specialists are set up to study problems, for example of work structuring, shift work, and non-functional differences between white and blue collar workers. It was remarkable that though industrial psychologists were normally founder members of such groups, occupational physicians were not. This exclusion seemed in the main to be determined by the doctor's lack of interest in contributing to the solution of problems outside his immediate work area and specialism.

It was noted that this dependence upon specialists, and their relationships with other parts of the organisation, became obstacles to progress in themselves. The specialist could often be instructed to examine a question perceived by the superior, whether or not that question was real, or of relevance to those whose situation came under scrutiny. The top manager might ask the Personnel Director to carry out a detailed study of an acute problem. The study would be conducted with considerable expertise, though perhaps without the participation of those most concerned; a detailed report would be prepared and submitted, only to arrive after the acute problem had been resolved. The report would be consigned to a filing cabinet without further attention.

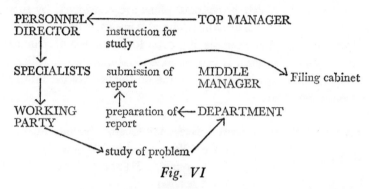

Fig. VI

In Italy, the situation seemed to be different. There too doctors, psychologists, and other specialists were included in membership of the Personnel Department, but unlike the Dutch model that department often had very poor links with either management or union, or sometimes within itself. In the Fiat factory, for instance, where paternalistic care for employees has been developed to include housing, hospitals, family medical care, and so on, the occupational physicians have virtually no communication with those looking after the family. A man falling ill at work will cease to be the concern of the occupational physician as soon as he goes home or to hospital, and that doctor plays no part at all in the care of the employee until he comes back to work on the recommendation of his family physician, who also works for Fiat!

Elsewhere the function of the personnel department tended to be action in the field of present occupational capacity, and rarely was there any influence by the personnel department on the development of long term commercial or organisational plans. The latter responsibility might rest with a Planning Department who might advise the Managing Director concerning long term plans, with little or no contribution from other areas of the business.

In one instance, it was the medical department which became involved in the criticism of an unrealistic plan so devised, and it was the company doctor who found himself in a position from which it was possible to insist upon the participation of the patients/employees concerned. The experience gained by the management team from this episode resulted in a new approach to problems, in which provisional plans are considered by those likely to be involved before the proposal is implemented.

Sweden is another example of greater formalisation of structure than is usual in Britain. It was possible to estimate the number of groups or specialists likely to be found on the basis of the number of people employed.

Company	Union	Joint Committee	Nurse & Personnel Adviser	Occu- pational Doctor	Social Worker	Psychol- ogist
1 employee	X					
25 employees	X	X				
500 employees	X	X	X			
2,000 employees	X	X	X	X		
4,000 employees	X	X	X	X	X	
10,000 employees	X	X	X	X	X	X

Partly perhaps influenced by the events and reactions to the national Mental Health Campaign in Sweden, a representative from that country proposed that, in time, medical staff might be employed jointly by unions and management in the future in order to "remove them from the arena of dispute".

British examples of the organisation of occupational medical service were quoted, in which the doctor reported to the Managing Director, though he might work very closely with the personnel department and contribute effectively to the formation of policy. It was noted that by becoming involved in general problems of the business, his own specialism might become diluted to the detriment of the quality of his specialist advice. He would also risk becoming an organisation man, and of being perceived as a committed manager rather than as an impartial professional. There was a particular need for renewal of medical expertise, perhaps to be derived from interaction with junior colleagues.

Consideration of the doctor's role has significance for all the other specialists, in that successful activity results from a subtle blend of personality and organisation. The hierarchy of the medical profession lent point to the importance of humility as an essential ingredient of team work. Only willingness to work in a team, and the recognition of the expertise of others, could lead to effective co-operation and communication between different disciplines.

Experience has shown that if less is said and listening is more attentive, communication flows upwards, as well as down the organisational chain. Frustration of attempts to comment upon the work being done is a stressor, and the resulting stress might otherwise be reduced by participation of all hierarchical levels concerned in the problems that confront them. This freeing of communication no more results from the stroke of a pen than does any other change of attitude. In creating conditions which permit two-way flow of conversation, no longer to be interpreted as "answering back", psychologists and doctors enjoy the particular advantage of the special place and responsibility they may have in the organisation. More than anyone else, they can behave in a way which demonstrates to others that gateways can be created which lead to new systems of communication, and so relating the outcome not only to greater efficiency, but to significant reduction of frustration and stress. Only if communication is so free can many problems be set in their true context.

The manager's filing cabinet might not be so full of unused information if the request for expert help could come from and include those concerned with the problem. Certainly less specialist time would be wasted, and the theoretical conclusions reached might well have more practical effects if those concerned had an opportunity to interpret and comment upon the information presented. The proposal to be implemented might then be perceived as the product of those who have to carry out the plan, and they would have a stake in ensuring that the plan should work.

There was a striking similarity of view concerning problems that arise in organisations, and the possible resolution of those difficulties, despite the wide range of nationalities and disciplines represented in the Windsor discussion. All were agreed that managers and those managed need education, so that they might become aware that someone is suffering stress, understand the individual's capacity to accept stressors, and realise that the sharing of commitment to an objective may reduce frustration and stress, if only temporarily. Moreover, the organisation as it is perceived by the individual is the cause of stress within him, so that it may not be valid to assume that because management has made an effort to reduce stress, that that attempt will be perceived as such by subordinates. On the other hand, there is a parallel with psychotherapy here, in that a tendency towards neurotic behaviour may result from the repression of what the ego does not want to know. This tendency is countered by participation by that person, who is supported while he lives through the confrontation with that which he would otherwise suppress.

Personality has already been mentioned. It may be thought obvious, but nevertheless does not seem to be sufficiently recognised, that the effectiveness of the organisation depends upon the personalities of those filling the various roles. If the medical officer in industry does not want to become involved in general problems, there is no point in organising the medical department with such participation as a major objective. From this particular example, confirmation if it were necessary could be derived for a general principle still obscure in many parts of industry. Technologists may not have the ability to manage; Research and Development may be led by a man without technical education; and the best craftsman may not be the potential foreman when his present superior leaves or is promoted.

10

Behavioural Science

IN 500 BC a Greek historian noted that the slave labour forces in Egypt were guarded by soldiers who were unable to speak their language, and who thus were immune to entreaty or corruption. It is significant that the importance of communication was recognised, and that the work force was organised on a military basis.

The command structure of industry in the eighteenth and nineteenth centuries was largely based upon the same military model, perhaps because that was still the most common example of larger work groups. Attitudes to communication were not so malevolent, but ignorance and greed led to almost as poor a quality of communication. Understanding of physical capability was deplorable to the extent of *reducing*, by Act of Parliament in the early nineteenth century, the minimum age of children working in industry to eight years. Soon afterwards, a Select Committee decreed that driving pulleys should be far enough from the ceiling to allow a child caught in a drive belt to go over the top and so come down again to the floor, rather than to be crushed to death against the ceiling!

Despite the activities of reformers, almost comparable ignorance persists into the twentieth century. One would have thought that sufficient had been learned about long hours of work in the last century to prevent abuse in this, but as late as 1917 it was noted with concern that despite increasing the hours of munition workers, production did not go up. For motives related more to the war effort than to a concern for people, a study was commissioned and published by the Industrial Fatigue Research Board. It was suggested that fatigue could be classified under three headings, and the committee reported that "Scientific management is fundamentally a problem of industrial fatigue, almost wholly confined to the nervous system, and its direct and indirect effects. . . ." "There is no obvious sign of nervous fatigue, and the man himself may be unaware of it, despite a diminishing capacity for work."

As post-war depression settled upon Britain, fatigue faded from the limelight, and despite some attention since, there are still people who expect—or are expected—to work for hours approaching, or even exceeding the sixty hour maximum demonstrated more than half a century ago.

In 1927 the Western Electric Company studied the effects of improved lighting in its factory in Hawthorne, Chicago. Elton Mayo examined the unexpected and unexplained results which were :—

1. that in three departments studied, erratic improvement in production was not related to the change in illumination
2. that when individuals were studied, both the "control" and "experimental" individuals showed the same degree of improvement.

In an experiment to explain those results, he asked two girls who were already friends to choose four others with whom to work in a newly designed, well-illuminated relay room. The experiment was in thirteen phases : —

1. A period of observation in the old department (2 weeks)
2. Moved to new room. No change in hours worked (5 weeks)
3. Eight weeks of piecework
4. Two rest pauses of five minutes each, in the morning and afternoon
5. Morning and afternoon breaks lengthened to ten minutes
6. Introduction of six five-minute rest periods in the day
7. Snacks provided as well
8. Total working day reduced by half an hour
9. Normal day further reduced by another half hour, i.e. one hour less work each day.
10. A switch back to the conditions of period 7
11. No Saturday working

12. Re-run of periods 1, 2, 3, with two hours extra work per day
13. Re-run periods 7, 8, 9 and 10

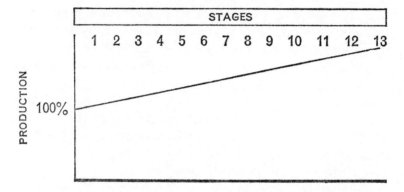

Throughout the whole period of the experiment lasting for over a year, there was an increase of 30 per cent in production, which was not reversed by reverting to worse conditions.

Elton Mayo proposed four possible explanations for this unexpected result, and discarded three of them. Improved materials and method might have been factors, but there was no conclusive evidence that this was so, despite subsequent efforts to demonstrate it.

Relief from fatigue was rejected because of the poor and sometimes adverse relationship between productivity and hours worked.

Reduction in monotony was rejected as an explanation because the typical "monotony curve" in production was absent, and because monotony was not a significant factor in the period before the study anyway.

The wage incentive was examined more closely in a second experiment, but applied in the absence of the other conditions, caused less than half the increase produced by the first experiment.

Mayo concluded that there was evidence of "an unexpected but highly potent variable in addition to other variables".

The girls involved in the first experiment expressed a sense of group identity, derived some satisfaction from being consulted, commented upon the new style of supervision which had displaced invigilation, and appreciated the attention of senior management as much as the changes in the pattern of work. Though other experiments were carried out, it is the one just described that is most famous. In the simplest terms, perhaps the fact that somebody *cared* was fundamental to the changes noted. Certainly the "Hawthorne effect" refers to this observation.

Obviously advances in psychology and psychiatry were being made in the orthodox medical field for many years before that experiment. Mesmer had treated patients for psychiatric disease in groups in the nineteenth century, and others were slowly developing this technique. Understanding of individual drives was dawning, and formalised attempts were being made to apply psychology to particular situations.

In the 1960's, McGregor in "The Human Side of Enterprise"[14] postulated two theories concerning work which he could see about him.

Theory X assumed that :

1. The average human being has an inherent dislike of work and will avoid it if he can.
2. Because of this human characteristic of dislike of work most people must be coerced, controlled, directed, threatened with punishment to get them to put forth adequate effort towards the achievement of organisational objectives.
3. The average human being prefers to be directed, wishes to avoid responsibility, has relatively little ambition, wants security above all.

Theory Y observed that :

1. The expenditure of physical and mental effort in work is as natural as play or rest.
2. External control and the threat of punishment are not the only means for bringing about effort toward organisational objectives. Man will exercise self-direction and self-control in the service of objectives to which he is committed.
3. Commitment to objectives is a function of the rewards associated with their achievement.

4. The average human being learns, under proper conditions, not only to accept but to seek responsibility.
5. The capacity to exercise a relatively high degree of imagination, ingenuity, and creativity in the solution of organisational problems is widely, not narrowly distributed in the population.
6. Under the conditions of modern industrial life, the intellectual potentialities of the average human being are only partially utilised.

McGregor suggested that "Theory Y" was true, and that it should form the basis for appropriate organisation and control of working groups.

There have been many attempts to develop understanding of human relationships, at many levels. The British War Office Selection Board procedure for identifying potential leaders attracted much attention from non-military organisations after the second World War, and from it have been developed two particular "experiential" courses referred to elsewhere in this book.

The introduction referred to a difference between cognitive and experiential learning. Cognitive learning is that derived from reading and objective observation. Experiential learning differs in that a planned experience of the student is the subject of study, with help from someone who interprets for him what is happening. The experience may be structured, in the sense that there is a definite programme of experience; or it may be unstructured to allow the student an opportunity to see how he and others in a group contribute to the development of a situation in which their own behaviour is analysed.

Typically, the Training Group, or "T"-Group as we refer to it, meets for at least a week, sometimes for a fortnight (see p. 122). After a Sunday social event, serving as an introduction to each other, the "T" group meets the following morning for the first time, and each member introduces himself with a short history, and a description of his job. Perhaps some members suggest a task that the group might do while others dissuade their colleagues from turning attention away from themselves, and towards a task. If the task is rejected, conversation flows sporadically about any topic under the sun, but members begin to notice who contributes, what the volume and quality of that contribution is, and how ready other members are to accept differing opinions. Typically, the "T" group tensions rise on the third very full day of discussions, because members have been in contact with each other for almost the whole of their waking hours throughout that time. On that third day, exasperation and impatience with one's fellows leads to pungent comment, which is returned.

This phase of activity has earned the jargon term "feed back", or the reflection of one's own behaviour in the comment of others. This process can be very painful, because many people have never heard what others think of them, often because opportunities to find out have not occurred, or have been avoided. In the "T" group situation such "feed back" may be expressed emotionally or with objective candour. Sometimes the process affords an opportunity to consider the difference between criticism and attack, and sometimes it is the commentator whose style is criticised by the group, who may feel that the criticism he expressed is not valid, not deserved, or is maliciously expressed.

It is in regard to this feedback that two schools of Training Laboratory can be identified. In one, criticism develops unchecked by the trainer, and may lead to concerted and sometimes cruel attack upon one member of the group by all his fellows. In the other school, some attempt is made, however arbitrarily, to set a limit to the degree of exposure to attack, while yet not preventing feedback altogether.

Because there is no structure, and because there is often a subtle inference that members are expected to perform a "spiritual striptease", discussion can range over a wide range of topics, and sometimes very deeply into some of them. Basic personal assumptions of individuals are questioned by other members of the group, and perhaps for the first time the individual questions some of his own. Questions of morality, religion, ethics, relationships with families, together with more obviously commercial topics as discipline and integrity attract attention. At the end of the experience, personality is rarely altered in type but it has certainly developed or modified in its expression. In a strange way, members emerge with relationships which would have taken decades to develop otherwise in neighbours or colleagues, and the experience leads to a greater awareness of the possible interpretations of the words and actions of others.

The Managerial Grid is another widely used method of management training. It has some of the elements of a "T" group experience, in that there is syndicate work leading to appraisal of individual members' styles, but it otherwise differs greatly in having tasks, targets, and critiques designed to hammer home the lesson of the Grid concept.

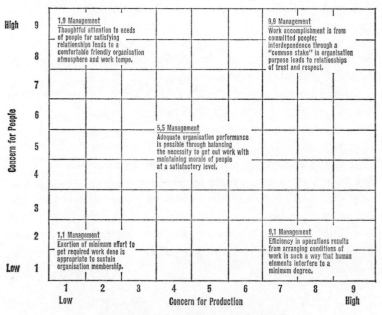

Fig. VII The Managerial Grid

The diagram expresses in the simplest terms the five management styles identified, and numerous exercises demonstrate the various styles. Throughout the week of the course, syndicates compare their own performance in the same terms, and at the end of the week, the performance and management style of each member of the syndicate is assessed by his colleagues under the main headings used in the exercises.

Many criticisms of either the Grid or "T" group technique

have been expressed from time to time. The significance of emotional breakdown is referred to elsewhere, but it is worth mentioning less serious but important problems here. There appears to be a compulsion on those suggesting participation in these courses that they should refrain from any attempt to convey what happens on the course to the candidate before he sets off. No attempt is made to prepare him for what will undoubtedly be a profound experience, and sometimes what reassurance there is, is ineptly expressed. In one management team, the first woman to go was reassured by a colleague—"Don't worry about Thursday night". Until then, she had had no reason to assume that there was anything to worry about on any night. The detailed prework sent to the candidate before attending a Grid course is intended to convey what he should expect, as well as being essential groundwork for the course.

Another topic already mentioned is that of "spiritual strip-tease". While no one actually states an expectation, there is nevertheless an inference which no one attempts to dispel, that the more the individual exposes himself, the more benefit he will derive. Anyone setting off on one of these courses should be told before he goes that he himself sets the limit on his personal privacy and that that limit will be respected by others. If no such assurance can be given, because it would not reflect the norm of that particular training laboratory, the candidate should be made aware of the possible pressures upon him.

Absenteeism

THE preceding chapters have set a theoretical framework, and have described briefly the stresses caused and encountered in real situations. There is mention of "political" attitudes to psychology, and to fears of the "manipulation" of individuals, in Chapter 13. Many of the processes referred to can be exemplified in the discussion of absentee behaviour.

It is common to refer to absenteeism as "The English Disease". In fact, absenteeism is a phenomenon of increasing importance in all industrialised communities. No attempt will be made here to establish a league table of those countries with the worst records, but much of what follows, though described in a British context, will be valid in other countries.

Absence from work can be attributed to holidays, to leave with or without permission, and to "sickness". Only the last will be examined here. It can be assumed that the longer the period of absence, the greater the objective evidence of incapacity for work. In most cases absence for a third or subsequent week in any one period is due to disabling illness, whether mental or physical. Periods of days, up to a total of a single calendar week may very often be due only partly to a demonstrable illness, the disease usually being trivial and rarely disabling, but nevertheless a "trigger" for a decision by the sufferer not to go to work.

Custom has led to the formalisation of a bureaucratic system of obtaining evidence to support the contention that the absentee is or was sick. In days gone by, when labour was plentiful, a man's job was secure only if he could provide a certificate, and the doctor would assist his patient by endorsing the latters' claim that he was ill, and so unable to work. More recently, as people's sophistication increases, so does their awareness of "not feeling well".

Some years ago "sickness" would have meant a moderately severe infection or considerable pain, but together with improvement in treatment, a lower threshold of discomfort and improved education cause modern patients to complain earlier. Thus while the longer term certificate still supports a contention identical to that of long ago, the short spell of absence is a phenomenon of modern times; so much so that it is more appropriate today to think of absence attributed to sickness as being two problems, not one. Longer term absence is a problem for doctors; absenteeism for periods of only a few days, up to a maximum of a week, although attributed to sickness, is a behavioural problem of interest to everyone, whether managing or managed, and only partly a medical matter.

The majority of those concerned in this problem have anxieties caused by the threat of change. All will be tempted to assume that because certificates have always been obtained, they have always been valid, and will continue to be so. For their part doctors will resent very much the implication that the short term certificates they issue merely endorse their patient's claim that he is unwell, rather than express an expert opinion. The patients in turn will consider their doctor to be inconsiderate if he refuses to issue a certificate to endorse their word; and will feel themselves to be at the mercy of employers if they appear without "a note".

Each fears the other's change of attitude, the doctor fearing the confrontation required if he refuses the note, or the loss of a patient, or the loss of father figure or even professional status; the patient feeling unable to challenge the system, having no advocate, or having to explain directly to his superior why he has been away without the doctor's note which has become a talisman for his protection. Certification becomes a socially acceptable excuse, though all concerned *know* that total incapacity is not the point at issue, even though they will not admit it.

Should it be possible to overcome the fear of the change itself, it becomes easier to consider short term absence objectively.

There is a great bulk of evidence available concerning withdrawal from work. Within the last decade, no less than four pamphlets dealing exclusively with the subject have been published by the Industrial Society, the Department of Employment, and the Office of Health Economics. A Symposium on "Absence Attributed to Sickness" led to a publication by the Society of Occupational Medicine.[15] Leaders have appeared in both the medical and the lay press, and still short term certificates survive!

In yet another attempt to get the message across, a selection of quotations follows which ought to convince someone. These quotations may lead the doctor to stop issuing short term certificates, and patients may be influenced enough to cease demanding, much less paying for, short-time certificates.

"The problems of turnover and absenteeism can be studied together, since in some respects the small decision which is taken when the employee absents himself is a miniature of the important decision he makes when he quits his job."[16] In 1955, Hill and Trist,[17] studying steelworkers in Sheffield, believed that the character of the decision to leave *finally* was essentially different from *temporary* withdrawal from work. Hill and Trist suggested three phases through which an employee passed after joining the company, and in the subsequent years. These phases were:—

1. The induction crisis;
2. The phase of differential transit;
3. The phase of settled connection;

and as such serve as useful headings under which to consider other studies.

The induction crisis: In the steelworks, this lasted for up to six months. During that time, the new employee would go "off sick" as a means of withdrawing temporarily from work, while adjusting to his new environment. This was considered to be the only method open to the newcomer, who might be unaware of, or reluctant to use, other means of coping with the new stresses.

That the element of personal choice rather than organic disability may be the major factor in such absence is an idea supported by several other writers. Hinkle and Wolf (1957)[18] found a relation between "illness clusters" and the individual's own perception of his life situation. More periods of absence occurred during times which were significantly more stressful to that individual, arising out of his relation to the total environment. Ekker, (1965),[19] in a study of 400,000 workers in three hundred firms in the Netherlands, suggested that the explanation for widely differing rates lay "less in the amount of sickness than in the reasons for either continuing to work or to stay away". De Groot (1965)[20] was even more explicit, "Experience has revealed that rates of sickness absence have practically nothing to do with differences in the state of health of groups of workers". In Britain, Chiesman (1957)[21] contended that staying away from, or return to, work did not depend on the start or cessation of a particular disease process, but on the patient's ability to adjust himself to the working environment.

The phase of differential transit : In the population studied by Hill and Trist, this period extended from the seventh to the thirtieth month of service. During this time the employee was considered to be both settling down, and availing himself of alternative methods of coping with unfamiliar stressors while adapting to the environment. In collating the figures upon which these phases are based, Hill and Trist considered serial months of service, not calendar months. Thus the "n"th month of service in every individual was compared, whether or not that "n"th month was the same calendar month. By this device, those authors claimed to flatten out possible seasonal variations in absence records which might be caused by epidemics occurring in winter months.

The settled phase : At the end of two and a half years, the periods of absence of the steelworkers had fallen to a level which was subsequently maintained. This the authors interpreted as evidence of adjustment to an environment which had become familiar. This tendency for absenteeism to fall as length of service increased has been noted before and since by other research workers. Their findings suggest that newcomers in factories are more liable to absenteeism than seasoned workers; sickness absence is highest in the employees staying only a short time; and, in the case of women employees, the absences from work drop as the term of employment increases, but the average *length* of absence gets higher.

Thus there seems to be evidence of an association between absenteeism and length of service. Is there any change in behaviour which could predict those who were going to leave? Buzzard and Shaw (1952)[22] considered that the workers they had studied took excessive sick leave before final departure from their firms.

The working population in Britain was described by Ennals (1969)[23] as consisting of one person in three who claims National Insurance at least once in any year. Among this section, one out of three claimed more than once. These figures do not include women who opt out of the national insurance scheme to depend upon their husband's contribution.

An earlier, closer look at a section of the general population by Ashworth (1956)[24] had shown that only 8 per cent of his patients accounted for half the total of days lost by those who went out to work in his general practice. Another study suggests that the individual's exising short term (especially one day) absence record could be the most informative datum on which to predict his likely future sick absence experience.

Among reasons other than sickness for absenteeism we must consider motivation as a possibly critical factor. Motivation of less skilled employees in the food manufacturing industry was recognised by the Economic Development Committee (1967) to be a particularly difficult problem, and it has been widely demonstrated that the more meaningful work can be made for the employee, the more powerful will be his motivation to return to work.

"All these problems—labour turnover, absenteeism, bad time keeping, low employee morale, and substandard work performance—can often be grouped together under one heading: the under-utilisation of human resources resulting from an individual withdrawing from work."[25]

From studies carried out in several continents, it must be concluded that the short-term absence certificate is a worthless piece of paper. Nonetheless it is demanded of individuals by employers, school authorities, and union sick pay schemes. Employers perpetuate the system by assuming that only absence not covered by a certificate is open to management action.

The manager has his fears about challenging the system, for how can he question a national insurance certificate? If he does question the certificate, he has to learn new techniques and attitudes for dealing with those in his care.

Ask any manager whether he is concerned about absenteeism, and the positive reply will mean that he is very much concerned with how many hands are available to him to do the work, but that he only expects "ritual" reasons for absence. While a manager's own superior accepts the manager's word that absence was due, for example, to domestic difficulties, or migraine, his subordinate Mrs. Smith, with three children, would be expected by the manager to provide a note to say that she had to stay at home with little Jimmy who had measles.

Some would say that this difference of approach is inspired by class prejudice, by political belief, or that it was merely typical of the unfairness of the manager concerned. Basically it may be the effect of a projection system—"We, the white collar workers, are expected to behave this way, they, the blue collar workers, behave like that". Simply stated, "us" and "them", (with each side considering themselves to be "us"), are denying that they belong to the same human race, with the same basic drives and needs.

If now we have reached an assumption that anyone may withdraw from work voluntarily for short periods, what should we do about it? The two groups most closely concerned, union and management, each considers the other to be "them", to have different drives, interests, and hopes, and to require coercion rather than understanding: if negotiations were to take place concerning a new approach to absenteeism, each delegation would not only have to watch its adversary, but would have to glance back at those it represents, to make sure that the negotiating group has continuing support from its constituency. The negotiators may behave in a way which they believe to be considered appropriate by those they represent and their antagonists. Each side adopts an aggressive/defensive attitude, which makes it very difficult for either side to say simply "we both know that 'x' is so, for 'y' reasons, and the options for dealing with the problems are 'z'." Each side spends time displaying to the other side and to its constituency, that the opponents have to be forced to recognise each point, rather than to accept the obvious. Much more negotiating effort is taken up in establishing the status and rights of the parties concerned, than in dealing with the problem that confronts them. Even before any meeting takes place such attitudes obscure the view of the problem to be discussed, because the various parts of the argument are reduced to mere bargaining counters in a win/lose confrontation, in which compromise rather than understanding is the objective.

If short term absenteeism were the problem, the basis for discussion might be the following points :

1. Periods of up to a week are not due to sickness, do not require a note, and do not qualify for sick pay.
2. Real disability could be compensated more generously, either in terms of more sick pay per week, subsequent to the second week in any period, or as a longer entitlement to sick pay, beginning at an earlier point in service.
3. Superior/subordinate relations should be such that an explanation by the returning employee that he was now better after 'flu should be acceptable directly by the manager concerned.

Now consider the approach of each side to such proposals :

The union must know that the first proposition is true, but how can they be seen to accept a proposal to reduce workers' benefits from the employer, and how can they themselves disqualify their own members from union sick pay for the first week ? They will probably continue to assume that the employer will victimise the absentee who does not produce a "note", or alternatively they will consider it a "diabolical liberty" for the manager to enquire directly why the subordinate has been away.

On the management side, there may be anxiety about the unions' likely demand to offset the loss of sick pay in the first week; there will be fear that junior managers may provoke a strike by ineptly refusing sick pay, and there will be unwillingness to provide time for management training in the understanding and control of absentees; there will be a wish to put the whole problem in the hands of medical staff "whose job it is to cope with sickness"! And in all probability there will be an expectation that the more generous system will be abused.

To some extent, the last two uncharitable paragraphs caricature union and management behaviour. But if both sides were to study the problem itself, and not the risks to their status inevitable in such a negotiation, something like the following appreciation of the problem might emerge (based on Raffle) :[26]

Repeated short absences may be caused by established underlying illness which cannot be improved. Management has to decide whether the unsatisfactory record is acceptable on the basis of the age, length of service, or other circumstances of the employee concerned. The union has to decide whether the "brother" deserves special consideration, in order to be allowed to do jobs outside his normal demarcation lines, and whether his "brothers" are to give him a hand with the heavier or more demanding work, or excuse him from it altogether.

In such a case, both sides may have to share the burden of deciding that the disability may be so grave and permanent that the employee should be under the care of some State or social agency. If he is to be retained, it must be as part of an attempt to employ him constructively for his own needs, insofar that they can be reconciled with those of the employer. He should not be retained in any job merely because neither side will recognise the significance of his condition to the productivity and quality of life of the community as a whole.

Underlying illness discovered spontaneously, or as a result of objective assessment, may be possible to improve so that the individual is restored to health and enabled to make an appropriate contribution to the society of which he is a part. That may be interpreted as a manipulation of the individual, but it is no more than a statement of fact. While the individual deserves due dignity, consideration, and compassion, he derives them ultimately from the society to which he has himself contributed. Conflict of interest is not inevitable, so that with the patient's consent, the health services, the employer, and the union can vigorously co-operate to restore the patient to health.

Some repeated absences may be due to social or family reasons, and the employers' role here may be to help the employee directly or to indicate an outside agency particularly qualified to help with a specific problem.

There remains that group of people whose absence behaviour has no evident pathological or social cause. Very often, the person concerned is not aware of his own absence record, and might see at once why such a record becomes unacceptable to an employer. Should the absence record not improve, he either leaves or is dismissed, because he is in the wrong job, with the wrong people, or is unwilling to share the work of his fellows.

It is this last mentioned group that demands most understanding. The people themselves must be enabled to examine and express their reasons for absence, and to be understood with appropriate compassion. They should not be forced to seek refuge in a meaningless bureaucratic ritual, which sweeps the real problem under the carpet. Those to whom they express dissatisfaction must learn to accept their right to complain, and their reasons for doing so. Both sides must seek remedies in terms appropriate to the real situation.

Perhaps we all fit into one or other categories at different times and certain conclusions become apparent : those who take sick pay "entitlement" because it is there might be recognised as taking extra holidays, so directing proper attention to holiday entitlement rather than to "sickness"; those who take "basic" days off and yet earn overtime might be seen to be doing so, not only by their management, but by their colleagues, who earn overtime more directly, and after more work; and those really ill might derive greater benefits from state and private schemes relieved of the burden of paying the man who decides not to work.

Above all, those who design the work would have to pay more attention to the satisfaction of those performing the various tasks necessary in modern industry.

A Company Campaign

Philips Electrical Industries in Holland produce a wide variety of electrical and electronic equipment. There are about 80,000 employees in the Netherlands of whom half work in Eindhoven. While there is no organised all-embracing programme for mental health, a great deal of work is done on personnel management and these activities have important preventive aspects.

Personnel management could be defined as the collection of efforts, projects and programmes meant to keep in harmonious balance the individual with his needs and disabilities on the one hand, with the social system, its demands and possibilities on the other. Personnel management aims at an optimal relation between the employee and the industrial organisation in the hope that primary prevention may be successful against stress both for the individual and the group. Activities meant to help the individual to function in the industrial organisation include selection, introduction and training, and different departments have responsibility for these topics.

In organisation and re-organisation there are efforts to change or to improve the systems, to reflect trends in standards of contemporary society as a whole, of which the industrial organisation is a sub-system. One example of such organisation is the structuring of work along more modern lines.[27] This is at present one of the largest programmes in personnel management in Philips, and has many consequences for the organisation. It started in 1963 and it is still developing in many departments. Projects are advised by psychologists, and socio-economic experts.

Other activities focused on the social system to improve its function for the individual include research on shift work and on morale of groups and departments, research into sickness absence, counselling in reorganisation projects, and ergonomics.

Just as important as restructuring the organisation is the problem of consolidation in order to keep it up to date. Man needs some continuity and stability in his environment to enable him to adapt to its changes. An example of this consolidation would be labour agreements which run for more than a year.

For many employees the measures of normal personnel management, with its preventive aspects, is sufficient but there always will be a group of employees for whom it is not enough. Their adaptational qualities are not adequate to cope with the demands of the system, and they will develop complaints and ill health.

Even in a well managed organisation, stressful situations cannot be prevented. For some employees, with an already delicate personal balance, stress occurs earlier than for others. Many of these employees will develop complaints about their health for which they seek help. The doctor is a time honoured institution to go to if personal, confidential aid is needed. This will invite many to "translate" whatever bothers them consciously or unconsciously into physical complaints. A recent investigation showed that one third of the complaints to general practitioners did not have any organic cause; one third were acute respiratory diseases; and one third were caused by more classical physical diseases.

But the person to whom the employee turns is almost chosen by chance. It could be the family doctor or the occupational medical officer, but the employee might turn to a social worker, or a personnel manager, or a psychologist, or a representative of his union. Whoever he turns to, he cannot be sure whether he will get adequate assistance; or whether the relation between his complaining and the psycho-social stress causing his trouble will be recognised.

Often, the tension, problems, complaints and sickness absence remain and the condition of the patient probably develops from bad to worse.

If the patient is in medical channels a series of physical

examinations is likely to follow, maybe consolidating the patient's belief in a "difficult to cure" somatic disease; maybe strengthening the conviction of his manager that "nothing is the matter". With a development like this, a new vicious circle of stress, misunderstanding and threatened self-esteem is set in motion.

A development like this is not imaginary. Psycho-social problems and their consequences are not easily understood. They are time-consuming to discover and often the patient himself has his resistances to uncovering his "weaknesses". Even when the patient and his doctor know what is causing all the trouble, it will often be difficult to alter the life or work situation to diminish the stress.

Developments in the medical and human sciences are tending to see the individuals and his environment as one entity. The experts, however, all with their own specialisation on different aspects of the life situation of an individual, have not been prepared (or trained) to operate as one entity. Co-operation is hampered by many barriers, which we can call "structural" in the sense that there are "proper channels" and "chains of command". Problems may be :

1. the expert knowledge of stress and psycho-social problems is not present in the field,
2. the "desired" experts are present, but they lack time to co-operate successfully,
3. even if the intention to communicate about an individual patient is present, the communication channels are not,
4. the training of the experts is insufficient for making co-operation rewarding. The psychologist, the social worker the personnel manager, the occupational medical officer, the general practitioner, have often a vague idea about the possibilities and capacities of the professional training of the others. They are not trained to understand each other, which makes it also impossible to refer a patient successfully because he does not fit into the "frame of reference" of the individual expert concerned.

Since not only mental but health care in a wider sense is endangered by difficulties in the understanding, communication and co-operation of experts, an attempt to improve the conditions is being developed in the medical department of Philips.

At the beginning of 1971 an automated information and communication system of medical data on individual persons started its output. With the aid of this on-line computer system it is hoped to help eliminate—amongst other things—administrative barriers, isolation of specialised experts, loss of essential data necessary for appropriate diagnosing and treatment of a person, and needless repetition of examinations caused by bad communication.

The main aim of this Medical Information and Communication System (MICOS) is to develop a Medical Archive for each person. For this, the medical and social experts share responsibility. By consulting the data bank immediate details are available of an individual's medical history, personal data, medical essentials, registration of contacts with medical or social experts, biometric data, and a register of diagnosis of absenteeism. All these facts will in future be directly available at the moment a patient appears before a doctor or before any other expert belonging to the team responsible for this person's health care, so that a patient can have contact with a complete team of health experts. This team will differ from person to person, depending upon the need of the patient.

Optimal information and communication are not enough. The experts will have to use and integrate the information about other aspects of health care, before the system is of any use for the patient. Another condition to work on is therefore the attitude of the experts to a system new to them, which will develop gradually when the possibilities of the system become clear to the participants and less threatening both to the patient and to the expert.

The impact of the automated system on the medical organisation will be great. To prevent stress symptoms in the health organisation itself, and to help the organisation adapt to the computer system, "change agents" are present. A sociologist and two psychologists are participating in the project team and are coaching system engineers and medical staff.

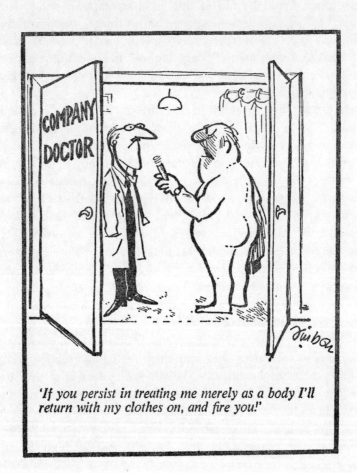

'*If you persist in treating me merely as a body I'll return with my clothes on, and fire you!*'

13

A National Campaign

IN Sweden, to a greater extent perhaps than in any other country the structural change within society, the urbanisation process, rapid technical developments, automation and rationalisation have all contributed to change man's living conditions and increase the psychological strains on the individual.

Problems at the place of work have taken on a very special importance during recent years. The individual is confronted with regrouping within companies, changing places of work, and moving from the country to new urban areas. Everywhere the tendency is toward a system of large companies where the old groups are broken up and where meaningful continuity becomes obscure. For the individual, anonymity in the midst of a crowd is becoming an increasing reality.

This is a development which can be explained in economic and technical terms and it has been a prerequisite for the rapid increase in the Swedish standard of living. But it has also had negative consequences in the form of increased stress, uncertainty, insecurity and isolation, and has led to an increase in both psychological and psychosomatic illnesses such as ulcers, heart ailments and high blood pressure. This is the background to the drive for "Mental Health at the Place of Work" which is being conducted by Folksam's health organisations and institutions.

Folksam is a Swedish insurance company which has invested a great deal of time and money in the investigation of events which affect policy holders. In 1961 the company investigated accident risks in team sports, and inspired sport organisations in the discussions of how sports injuries might be prevented. In 1962 another investigation focused on the relationship between the human being, the machine, the environment, and the need for physical exercise. Being concerned with Man, Machine, Milieu, and Motion, the investigation became known as the "4M Drive" (as part of that activity, 63,000 study groups of up to a dozen people came into being).

There is no doubt that the 4M Drive aroused interest in ergonomics, and cleared the path for more active study than had previously been possible. But in doing so, the whole question of gauging the needs of the individual against changing work requirements became more significant, and preparations were made for a programme to be launched in 1968 on the topic of "Mental Health, a campaign for increased understanding and solidarity within working life". This programme was based upon the existing structure of study groups which had formed for the previous exercise. Where there was no such group, safety or other works committees became involved in discussion.

An "organisation committee" with representatives of the collaborating organisations led the campaign. Its members included representatives of different professions, manual and clerical workers, weekly and monthly paid staff, company doctors, staff managers etc. Under the organisation committee was a secretariat within the Folksam Insurance Company which had the responsibility for planning and organising the campaign, and in order to make it possible for so large a population to study the subject, two books were commissioned—"Work and Mental Health" by Erland Mindus,[28] and "Individual Personality and Human Environment" by Curt Amark.[29] Later, a correspondence course was made available.

The ultimate goal of all this activity was to make everyone more conscious of his own role in the work situation, and to broaden tolerance of fellow workers. However, in the spring of 1969 a critical reaction was started by students from some sociological, psychological and medical departments. They were opposed to the concept of mental health and adjustment as well as to the goals of the campaign.

The attacks were first concentrated on the authors of the basic books, but later switched to those research departments which were mainly concerned with sociological studies of working conditions and the relationships on the job. Later the organisers suspected that the opposition was politically inspired by groups with an intense dislike for the establishment! The mental health campaign as well as occupational medicine were criticised as acting on behalf of the employers in order to manipulate the employees to accept present conditions.

Though clearly intended to bring the campaign to a stop, the attacks had the opposite effect. People started to discuss these problems and a number of disputes and "wild cat" strikes gave an additional spur to observe and discuss the effect of the psychological atmosphere on places of work. Stress, mental health aspects of work, the meaning of work, alienation of the employees and such problems were discussed by the public at large, as well as by the discussion group themselves. An estimated number of 16,000 people have been active in the study groups, and a psychological consultant has been engaged to make some measurements of the change in attitudes resulting from this national campaign.

It is, however, doubtful whether a national mental health campaign could be mounted in the United Kingdom. Differences in the standard of living, the greater conflict between management and unions, the conflicts possible among a multiplicity of unions in the same industry, and perhaps most of all the different standard of education would seem to be major obstacles in the way of such an effort.

It is the experience of occupational physicians to be regarded as "tools of management". This attiude would present a particular problem in any British programme of education because (as in its Swedish predecessor) doctors and psychologists would be suspected of attempting to manipulate the attitudes of individuals to their work situation. What is more, the wider gap between employer and employed in the U.K. would be more likely to lead to bargaining about proposals—any campaign of this kind is almost certain to be regarded as a threat to some, for reasons which are psychological perhaps more often than political.

14

Management Development

IN one large British group of companies, it was realised some years ago that only a small proportion of managers who were said to have some potential, enjoyed access to, and the benefits of, a conventional management programme. Only a small budget was available for such training, so that the personnel department operating the scheme tended to make training proposals where they were most likely to be accepted.

More thorough performance appraisal of a wider spectrum of management emphasised training and development needs—and a recognition that the budget for training would have to be increased. The personnel department's role, it was then felt, should be directed less to nominating those requiring training, and more towards the assessment of outside training resources, or special assignments which would afford relevant experience opportunities. Career planning mechanisms were revised, as it became evident that many more managers than hitherto would be involved in the development of specific skills which would in turn improve the performance of the companies.

A management training centre was set up, and external activities were examined in depth. As many more people became involved, so the budget available was increased, enabling longer term plans to be made. Key people in related roles were selected for development, not so much in terms of individual potential as in supportive roles. These changes caused anxiety, particularly in the sense that those affected were uncertain of top management intentions. Several interpretations were placed upon events. "Clearly" some people were to be "developed" for promotion or transferred to other posts. Others were sure that everyone was to have his own performance increased. Some managers regarded the new programme as a test of their potential, or as an opportunity for personal growth, and development of new skills. Perhaps the older men regarded the programme as an attempt to prevent technical, managerial, or even spiritual obsolescence.

Needs which became apparent were those expressed by the individual himself, or those perceived by his superior. Succession planning was related to analysis of the skills necessary for current role descriptions. Moreover, comparison with the external world, awareness of new knowledge, and the recognition of failure to achieve operational goals suggested other needs. Confronted with these, training staff found it necessary to examine critically their own competence and acceptability. Training had to satisfy the trainee's perception of the needs of the business. The training staff had also to cope with problems arising from their own isolation from the business, while paradoxically maintaining that isolation necessary to ensure the privacy of performance and behaviour in those who took part in in-company training programmes.

As the training programme developed, management's view of training goals appeared ambiguous and required clarification, as did the criteria for selection of individuals for the various types of training available. There was evidence to suggest the need for more voluntary attendance and self-selection, and the "back home" situation had to be such as to allow the returning manager to exercise his new skills. This more participative management style, and the greater dependence on team work, were seen to require new and very different behavioural skills in social and interpersonal relations.

In in-company training programmes, substantial experience exists of the use of various types of process analysis and critique of individual and group performance in discussions, on cases and exercises. Typically these concepts are introduced, in a week's programme, using trainers to record at 15-second intervals the nature of the contribution being made (contributing ideas, summarising, criticising, for example) and the individual making it. The data may be given to the group anonymously for them to discuss and explore. Typically, attention is later focused on how well the group worked in solving the problems presented in cases and exercises, and in what helped and hindered. Participants' generated data is shared and discussed openly. Not infrequently standard interpersonal response questionnaires are used, the depth of the discussion being determined by participants rather than by the trainers.

These and similar, sometimes more direct methods to produce feedback to individuals in a "safe" situation, are frequently marked as high points of programmes by those who took part, sometimes in terms of personal insight on how the individual functioned in group working, sometimes in terms of helpful personal feedback, though on rare occasions feedback is felt as punishing and unacceptable.

Successful use has been made of Phase I of Blake's Grid seminars.[30] External research in another large unit had demonstrated modest but noticeable improvements in behaviour in real work situations. Subsequently most participants advocate re-use of the programmes, but two objections have been expressed. In groups composed of mixed levels of management the critique of performance and feedback to individuals less well trained and less able has been described as "hurtful" and "distasteful". And a point which applies to any type of training course was that the amount of pre-work, and participants' views of the importance of meeting intensive work programmes, have produced conditions of excessive fatigue and some stress in individuals, particularly if they were under stress before attending. Attempts are made to meet these objections, while the use of these programmes continues with in-company personnel trained in the methods by the originators.

More than half the people attending Training-Group programmes run in this country, Europe and in the U.S.A. report favourably on their experiences although the utility of certain parts of T-Group programmes is questioned, and one significant stress reaction has been observed.

The general strategy in the use of T-Groups is that they will be used on a small scale, preference being given to nominations of key people in roles highly concerned with organisation change. To the extent that it is possible to achieve this aim, only volunteers attend and certainly no individual is designedly selected "because he needs it". A high premium is placed on using institutions and programmes whose professional and ethical standards are high.

In no other area of management development activity are so many and such substantial concerns expressed about ethical and stress issues. Some common myths have been expressed :

"People are forced to talk about their private lives"
"You work all night"
"It's brainwashing"
"Breakdowns are commonplace"
"People lose their power to make decisions"

More realistic problems have, however, become apparent. The "Training Group" is not appropriate for people already under stress or psychiatric treatment, and certainly not for an unwilling attender. There are doubts about the morality of subjecting employees to an experience which may produce behaviour or attitude changes. The "back-home" situation at work may be an obstacle to the practice of new skill, and since the experience is not limited to specifically "work" problems, wives and families may find it difficult to readjust to change, or the fear of change, in husbands whose new personal insight sometimes enjoys less than adequate understanding.

A particularly important feature of T-Groups is the professional and ethical standard of the trainer. Broadly speaking there are two schools : one which intervenes in the discussion to protect vulnerable participants from unreasonable attack; and the other which will not intervene whatever happens, because such interference will modify what would otherwise be a sort of "natural" process of group dynamics.

As a result of training and development programmes similar to that just described, stress, conflict, and ethical issues of such development are increasingly understood, so that programmes are better tailored to reconcile personal and organisational needs.

At the Windsor seminar, a quotation from Mr. John P. Campbell and Mr. Marvin D. Dunnette, both of the Industrial Relations Center, University of Minnesota, made clear that two elements used to distinguish the T-Group from other training methods are the learning goals involved and the processes used to accomplish these goals.

Advocates of T-grouping tend to focus on goals at two different levels (Buchanan, 1965 : Schein & Bennis, 1965). Flowing from certain scientific and democratic values are several metagoals, or goals which exist on a very general level. Shein and Bennis mentioned five, which they asserted to be the ultimate aims of all T-Group training :

(a) a spirit of inquiry or a willingness to hypothesise and experiment with one's role in the world;
(b) an "expanded interpersonal consciousness" or an increased awareness of more things about more people;
(c) an increased authenticity in interpersonal relations or simply feeling freer to be oneself and not feeling compelled to play a role;
(d) an ability to act in a collaborative and interdependent manner with peers, superiors, and subordinates rather than in authoritative or hierarchical terms; and
(e) an ability to resolve conflict situations through problem solving rather than through horse trading, coercion, or power manipulation.

It is true that not all practitioners would agree that all T-Groups try to accomplish all of these aims, but they are sufficiently common to most discussions of the T-Group method that they can be listed as the direct or proximate outcomes desired. The list is drawn from a variety of sources (Argyris, 1964; Bradford *et al*, 1964; Buchanan, 1965; Miles, 1960; Schein & Bennis, 1965; Tannenbaum *et al*, 1961) :

1. Increased self-insight or self-awareness concerning one's own behaviour and its meaning in a social context. This refers to the common aim of learning how others see and interpret one's behaviour and gaining insight into why one acts in certain ways in different situations.
2. Increased sensitivity to the behaviour of others. This goal is closely linked with the above. It refers first, to the development of an increased awareness of the full range of com-

municative stimuli emitted by other persons (voice inflections, facial expressions, bodily positions, and other contextual factors, in addition to the actual choice of words) and second, to the development of the ability to infer accurately the emotional or noncognitive bases for interpersonal communications. This goal is very similar to the concept of empathy as it is used by clinical and counselling psychologists, that is, the ability to infer correctly what another person is feeling.

3. Increased awareness and understanding of the types of processes that facilitate or inhibit group functioning and the interactions between different groups—specifically, why do some members participate actively while others retire to the background? Why do sub-groups form and wage war against each other? How and why are pecking orders established? Why do different groups, who may actually share the same goals, sometimes create seemingly insoluble conflict situations?

4. Heightened diagnostic skill in social, interpersonal, and intergroup situations. Achievements of the first three objectives should provide an individual with a set of explanatory concepts to be used in diagnosing conflict situations, reasons for poor communication, and the like.

5. Increased action skill. Although very similar to No. 4, this refers to a person's ability to intervene successfully in inter— or intra—group situations so as to increase member satisfactions, effectiveness, or output. The goal of increased action skill is toward intervention at the interpersonal rather than simply the technological level.

6. Learning how to learn. This does not refer to an individual's cognitive approach to the world, but rather to his ability to analyse continually his own interpersonal behaviour for the purpose of helping himself and others achieve more effective and satisfying interpersonal relationships."

Earlier in this chapter reference has been made to some "myths" about T-Group and Grid Training. There have, in fact, been some breakdowns on such courses, which led to informal meetings, at and following the Windsor conference, between several doctors in various companies, some personnel managers, and a psychiatrist with extensive experience of management training method. Although originally directed to the study of T-Groups and Grids some observations were made which can appropriately be applied to any training course whatever its type or purpose, and whoever it is that goes.

One viewpoint, for instance, was that the range of normal behaviour in groups was sometimes misunderstood by people who had not attended that form of training.

Some degree of anxiety, tension or withdrawal were quite appropriate emotional reactions for some members of a group, as that group worked through its task. Tears or silence alone were not evidence of incipient breakdown but might be entirely appropriate, and possibly even valuable. Criticism even when frank and pointed was not to be confused with personal attack. The use of strong language towards an individual who persistently blocked his group's progress on its task was entirely understandable. Behaviour which in another setting might be embarrassing or discomforting may be sanctioned by such a group and not accompanied by individual distress.

It was generally felt that whatever the nominal position, no scheme of training could be entirely voluntary. As soon as the training is generally adopted individuals felt themselves under all kinds of pressure to conform. When outright refusal to attend was not respectable it could be replaced by passive resistance strategems. For example, initial acceptance of a place for a training experience was followed by an eleventh hour withdrawal on the grounds of a sudden rush of work.

Briefing for any management course can be combined with self selection. To be effective such briefing must be detailed and handled sympathetically. What is intended as a defusing operation should not itself become a stressful experience. The procedure recommended was a thorough briefing session designed by the candidate's manager where he has himself attended some form of sensitivity training, representatives of Personnel Department involved in the training programme, and the company doctor who has had experience of the form of training to be discussed.

The manager's role can be vital in explaining convincingly the expectations of training and its relevance to the departmental development. The manager must also play a part in encouraging a participant to set sensible work norms during training.

Large scale industry is, of course, in a unique position to undertake a research programme aimed at evaluating selection for T-Group courses. Predictions of performance and emotional response could be made and checked by what happened. Actual learning could be assessed from subsequent performance and progress.

As the largest group of casualties are of the exhaustion type, the prevention of fatigue is important in reducing the number of cases of breakdown. Fatigue is not directly and simply related to the number of hours worked. Account must be taken of other factors such as motivation, stress, competitiveness and the degree of support which individuals feel within their group. Nevertheless the setting of sensible norms is recommended.

This subject should be fully discussed at the briefing session, should receive attention at the beginning of the laboratory or seminar, and should be carefully watched by trainers throughout a course. In the case of Grids it is important that adequate time should be devoted to the preparatory tasks, and that this should not be compressed into a few days' concentrated work prior to arrival. Managers have a particular responsibility to ensure that subordinates about to depart for training are not overloaded with routine work.

At Windsor no firm conclusions were reached about trainer skills. Some Grid trainers are known to be inexperienced and to have had only very sketchy training, but these deficiences cannot be linked confidently with the occurrence of breakdowns. Insight sufficiently keen to perceive the very earliest signs of illness is a fairly rare personal attribute. Even experienced psychiatrists acting as consultants in groups had been taken by surprise.

It is desirable to draw trainers' attention to a phenomenon which has been observed in some cases of breakdown. Certain people become active beyond the group norm, discover the "mystic core of meaning" of group training and attempt to proselytise their companions. This type of magical thinking (which might at first masquerade as great insight) can well presage breakdown.

15

Courses for Doctors

IT is easy to teach doctors new methods of testing the functions of the cardiovascular system, or the treatment of cancer, the appropriate use of antibiotics, or operative techniques. However, it is difficult to teach a doctor how to conduct a talk with his patient—and it is even more difficult to enable him to teach others by telling him how and what to teach.

The initial difficulty is that with so many instruments available for measuring objective facts to a finite degree, dialogue with the patient has been reduced to a minimum. Even that minimum can be achieved by giving the patient a questionnaire simply to mark "yes" and "no". By this, objectivity is said to be even better guaranteed. A computer provides the final opinion, a crown of objectivity, because it precludes the possibility of a doctor making an error. For every diagnosis the pharmaceutical industry has a ready-made medicine which makes direct communication with the patient unnecessary.

Attempts are made to create awareness among the public by making brochures, posters, and films, and by giving lectures on special occasions, such as Mental Health Week. This may help, but the patient is as much in need of a sincere talk with his doctor as he was about a thousand years ago. Patients need to know more about themselves, their behaviour, and how to develop healthy relations with other people; and this is the basis for healthy communities.

The original meaning of the word "doctor", i.e. teacher, was forgotten long ago and this task, which is one which needs great knowledge, skill and personal involvement, is now generally relegated to a secondary role. While some doctors are naturally good teachers, training of medical officers to be able to teach mental health is dependent upon several factors. Obviously they must be well motivated to learn, and to be able to cope with psychological concepts. In any group, one or two who do not recognise frustration or mental hygiene and related topics can play havoc with study attempts by the rest of the group, all of whom may have to realise that they must "unlearn" attitudes taught at medical school, or who may indeed have passed through their career to date with no formal education in psychology at all!

The programme must be well designed and couched in practical terms. Theoretical learning has no priority, because from intelligent and emotionally mature graduates, discussion of an introduction to group dynamics may crystallise into a theme which becomes the basis for the whole course. Some of the difficulties encountered in training doctors became evident during a seminar attended by fifteen doctors, working in an Institute of Physical Medicine and Rehabilitation, and by several doctors working in industry. While the latter had a very good attendance record, the former continually found excuses for absence.

The discussion leader confronted the first group with the question "What interests you, and what does not, in this course." The group enthusiastically began to list those factors which discouraged them :

1. loss of income while on the course
2. no great interest in the subject
3. too heavy a workload anyway
4. no great future financial advantage to be gained from the course
5. a sense of inadequacy to cope with the subject
6. attendance required by their director

These disadvantages obviously outweighed the few advantages recorded :

1. desire for new knowledge
2. satisfaction to be gained from mastering a new field
3. a few members of the group saw a higher status resulting from a Master's degree.

The most interesting of all these points was the "direction" to be on the course. Some members of the Institute became aggressive, blaming their Director or others for exerting pressures upon them to attend. None of the group could understand why the Director had been so insistent, since he had never been so before. On the contrary, he had always been ready to listen to counter-argument, and to understand especially their personal problems.

The discussion leader asked for possible reasons for the Director's behaviour in insisting upon attendance at that particular course :

1. to raise the quality of professional work
2. to win further recognition for the Institute itself
3. to justify the Institute's use of funds, by having evidently specially trained staff
4. to build up a new research establishment
5. to increase the Director's own reputation in medical circles

When the fifth reason had appeared, one of the group realised that he had only then thought of the Director's personal reasons for sending him on the course, and discussion suggested that all members of the group were realising that their attitudes to the course were selfish, rather than related to others in their organisation, or the organisation itself. Each justified his original stand or his change of attitude by blaming others, but they all realised that they were avoiding the issue. Then they agreed that the course would be acceptable "if well organised", and this in turn led to explanation of why they had not replied constructively to letters they had received prior to the course, containing a draft programme.

Some weeks later, discussions were resumed, this time in the presence of the Director. His explanation for his "atypical" behaviour was that he had considered it necessary to send his colleagues on the course, because he feared that if he did not order them to do so, they would not have gone because of the amount of work already outstanding.

From all that had happened, the discussion leader was able to demonstrate principal motives, the conflict between them, the choice of the most satisfying, and the significance of what members of the group had experienced to their understanding of situations which occur in other circumstances.

It may surprise the reader to know that the seminar described above took place in Yugoslavia, and was composed entirely of doctors trained and working in that country. Experience in other countries is similar, and a particular problem exists in Britain, and those countries which have a similar curriculum of medical education.

When considering problems of industrial mental health, doctors often find that the medical model, on which they were trained to make diagnoses, is of limited use to the patient or to the organisation in which they work.

On this model, unpleasant feelings in the mind of the patient are liable to be assessed by the same diagnostic methods as are organic disorders of the body or the brain. An approach on this model is quicker and often easier than one based on other models, the findings are simpler to write up, and many patients prefer it.

A major limitation is that the patient may not be given the opportunity of discussing his emotional difficulties fully and of having his feelings understood. Doctor and patient may therefore find themselves at cross purposes, because the doctor is looking for manifestations of a recognisable psychiatric illness which can be treated by specific remedies, whereas the patient may be wanting help with his personal problems.

Two other models which are often more helpful are available to the doctor; the psychodynamic model, and the model of group dynamics.

When using the psychodynamic model the doctor is predominantly concerned to assess the patient's personality and his particular psychological problems and emotional needs. An approach based on this model takes longer than in the diagnostic model, is usually harder for the doctor, the findings are difficult to write up, but the immediate complaints also receive attention as being possible symptoms of deeper emotional problems. Many may be connected with personal or family difficulties unrelated to the patient's work but manifesting themselves there, as irritability, depression, or a decrease in the level of his efficiency.

However, there may be psychological problems in the

interaction between the individual and his working environment, and it is these problems which give rise to what is known specifically as "stress at work". Stress may arise from various sources. Technological changes may have altered the requirements of his job. The employee may have been over-promoted, or under-promoted, or the limits of his responsibility may be unclear.

Stress may also result from difficulties with other people at work : for example, strong feelings of rivalry or marked competitiveness in the pursuit of power may result in uneasiness or anxiety. Another major source of stress is difficulty in adapting to the culture of the particular organisation.

On the other hand it may be that it is the organisation itself which is in difficulty. The interactions within it of its social structure, its culture and the individuals it employs are bound to produce stress, and in an organisation, as in an individual, a certain amount is a necessary stimulus to achievement.

In general, there is an optimal level of stress for each organisation, as for each individual. Diminution is harmful, and such an organisation can easily become inefficient and the individuals in it institutionalised with an impoverishment of their personalities. When stress is excessive, however, it may reveal itself by such group symptoms as an increase in sickness absence, prolonged absence for each spell of sickness, absenteeism, or increase of accident proneness.

The use of the model of group dynamics helps the doctor to consider the organisation itself as the patient. Towards the end of the last war, medical officers in some army units were required to submit to their divisional commanders weekly statistics on the health of their units. If the sickness rates for various illnesses consistently appeared to be above average, the commanding officer of that unit, not his medical officer, was held accountable.

It was considered that these figures were indices of the state of morale of the unit, which was in itself a reflection of the quality of the leadership, or management. When the relevant difficulties in the unit could be identified and resolved, an increase in morale of the unit was usually accompanied by a reduction in the incidence of sickness. Numerous concepts about health problems in organisations have, in the past 25 years, evolved and developed from this type of experience.

Which model should the doctor use?

There is no absolute answer; it depends largely on the way in which he sees his role with regard to his patient and to the organisation in which they both work. If the doctor sees himself as being predominantly concerned with individual episodes of illness, he will work more effectively with the first model. If the doctor sees himself as being more concerned with the psychological problems of the people in the organisation, he will base his assessments and therapeutic approach on the second and third models. If, however, the doctor sees himself not so much as a doctor to care for the individuals but more as an adviser to the whole organisation, he will then base his approach almost exclusively on the third model.

The model the doctor chooses will, however, also be determined by the character of the organisation in which he works and the attitude of the management to the doctor's role. In one place the doctor may be expected to limit his activities to helping the individual to adapt to the existing culture of the organisation, whereas in another he may be expected primarily to be involved in studying the dynamic nature of the organisation and the ways in which it may affect the individual.

In training a doctor to approach the problems of mental health in industry, it is useful to base the training on all three models, because it then enables him to ask such questions as: How much is the individual's disorder one where a specific medical remedy will bring relief? How much is it a symptom of pressures in the organisation, stemming from its social structure, its culture or the personalities of key personnel, about which advice to management may be appropriate?

Ideally one might say that the specific aims in training are to enable the doctor to identify the problems, to understand them on all three models, to learn how to organise appropriate treatment, and to develop his own expertise in training his managerial colleagues in their part in maintaining the mental health of the organisation.

Teaching, in the formal sense, can equip effectively a doctor to use the medical model, to recognise the patterns of psychiatric disorders and learn the physical remedies which may give relief. It is also possible to a certain extent, to teach, by formal methods, the principles of individual psychodynamics and of group dynamics.

A recent course in London of 12 lecture-discussions for Industrial Medical Officers was considered to be of considerable value, but there is a limitation in that the participants have to tolerate the frustration of accepting that what they can get from such a course is much less than they would wish.

This frustration arises directly from the fact that it is difficult to teach someone how to apply the principles of psychodynamics in his daily work or how, in practice, to increase his range of responses in situations in which his own feelings are aroused. Moreover, time is needed to assimilate these concepts and to acquire these skills.

A method of training which aims to help doctors to learn from their current experience in their work, is the ongoing seminar. In such a seminar eight to ten doctors meet regularly for one and a half hours a week with a psychiatrist trained in the techniques of leading such a seminar. It is preferable for all the participants to be of roughly the same level of ability, experience and sophistication.

The participants present case material from their current daily work, which is studied fully, with particular reference to their difficulties in managing the situation. Each participant is quite free to accept or reject any comments made in the seminar. After a few weeks the same doctor reports the progress of his case and this is discussed further. Thus, after a few months the seminar knows well, and is considering, several on-going cases.

There are numerous variations in the technique of running such a seminar. The technique employed by one British psychiatrist is based on keeping in mind five possible areas on which to focus the attention of the seminar, on one or more of which he may concentrate in any one session, depending on the circumstances.

1. The case material, with the doctor's assessment. This is

discussed by the seminar with particular reference to the patient's problems and needs.

2. The doctor/patient relationship. The doctor may, for example, be finding it difficult to tolerate the anxiety aroused in him by what the patient is saying, or by what the patient may be trying to make him feel. He may be finding it hard not to take premature action under the pressure of such anxieties. Similarly the doctor may feel himself being drawn into accepting the patient's viewpoint against his own critical judgement. He may find himself unable adequately to help patients to cope with their frustrations, or he may be in difficulty through not understanding the material.

3. The psychodynamics of the actual material being discussed, about which the seminar leader may teach. It seems, from experience, that teaching is more effective in a setting where participants are actively, at that moment, interested and involved in a problem. That has the advantage over formal lectures which may or may not be of interest at that particular time.

4. Further work which the doctor might do with the patient, further problems he might profitably try to clarify, further information he might elicit, and possible courses of action. Although the seminar can help to clarify the situation, each doctor must make, and be responsible for, his own decisions.

5. Problems within the seminar itself. Sometimes the seminar finds itself unable to proceed satisfactorily with its work task which is to study the various aspects of the material presented by the participants. Members may have feelings of rivalry with each other or with the seminar leader. Anxieties about certain topics may lead to an unconscious collusion between members not to pursue them further. Numerous situations may stir up feelings of aggression. The work task of the seminar may then be blocked until these conflicts themselves have been examined and resolved by those present.

It will readily be seen that numerous new experiences have to be faced and digested. For this reason participants should be prepared to attend for about eighteen months to two years (60 to 80 sessions). Although that is the ideal duration, participants sometimes find that under pressure of various requirements at work they can only commit themselves for 20 sessions and courses have been run on this basis. The work of such a seminar is considerably restricted but nonetheless some worthwhile results can be obtained even on this limited basis.

A particular type of seminar which can be extremely valuable is an interdisciplinary one to study the psychological aspects of problems of mutual concern.

Run on similar lines to those already described, a group of ten to twelve participants, consisting of three or four workers from each of three disciplines whose work overlaps, meet regularly with a psychiatrist. On-going seminars of this type have been run for G.P.s, psychiatrists, and social workers, and one based on the needs of an industrial organisation, such as a group consisting of managers, of personnel officers and of industrial medical officers, might be an acceptable and valuable training experience.

No one group is teaching the other, but the members of each group and the psychiatrist contribute from their respective viewpoints. Experience with this type of seminar has shown that there are certain difficulties in the initial stages because each professional group tends to be apprehensive of the other, often on the basis of competitiveness and rivalry. When these difficulties have been faced and worked through, the sharing of the thoughts and feelings of the different groups is an enriching experience for the participants.

Numerous seminars of these types have been run successfully for G.P.s, probation officers, social workers and psychiatric registrars. In these forms of training the strains on the participants can be considerable. It is often not at all easy to have to expose one's own psychiatric work for detailed scrutiny by colleagues, and marked pressure is frequently put on the seminar leader to change his approach and give practical guidance. It is also a strain to have to give up to a large extent a model of working on which so much of one's undergraduate and postgraduate education has been based, while simultaneously learning to work with other models which one hopes, but cannot be certain, will be more rewarding.

The doctor's ability to respond to these strains will depend not only on his desire to learn, but also, as in any process of learning, on his ability to tolerate the anxiety of uncertainty throughout the process of learning. It might be said that as well as whatever skills that are learned, a very valuable outcome is an increased ability to tolerate anxiety in his work. Eighteen months has been found, from experience, to be the shortest period of time for which a participant must attend a training seminar to give himself a reasonable chance to achieve this result.

A totally different approach to learning from current experience is when two doctors, from different specialities, work closely together to study individual cases from the viewpoints of their respective disciplines.

In a current experiment by the British psychiatrist already mentioned, he spends one afternoon a week working with an industrial medical officer in a large organisation. He is referred cases in which there might be psychological factors which he and the industrial doctor then discuss, sharing their views, which are based on the training and experiences of their different specialities. This is a mutual training experience, the industrial doctor learning about psychiatry, and the psychiatrist learning about industrial problems.

As in the seminar, the aim of the psychiatrist is not to teach the industrial doctor how to manage psychiatric problems in an industrial setting—the psychiatrist is not equipped to do so— but to help to clarify the psychiatric aspects so that the industrial doctor can feel himself more fully equipped to try to evaluate it by discussion, questionnaire, and perhaps also, as after a recent teaching course for industrial medical officers, by an examination paper.

The nature of further courses can then be determined by the views and needs of the participants.

16

Society's Role

ORGANISATIONS and individuals; groups varying in size from race, through nationality, religion, social class, and club to the few people who make up a working party or committee; and the community of which an individual is part, have all received attention, and the varying influences which operate have been sketched. Throughout, there has been a tendency to describe what is happening, and to explain why it should. When measures to prevent or remedy the causes of stress in individuals are concerned, the concept of "society" conveys more than a collective noun; the structure and aims of the community come to the foreground, while the size and organisation of the community serve only as a background.

Earlier, it was explicitly assumed that each human animal has some degree of responsibility for his actions. In some minds, responsibility is part of the function of an individual's soul. It may be helpful to regard the concept of "society" as if it were the soul of the whole community. In that sense, society's "spiritual" responsibility for all the people who form the "body cells" of the community will be considered here.

Despite considerable misgivings, it is possible to force through the pen the statement that economic systems of developed countries whether capitalist or not, do not vary very greatly in the benefits bestowed upon the great mass of people they affect. The United States is acknowledged as the world's richest country and, though less now than before, proudly claimed to be a land of opportunity. But where are the opportunities for its four million unemployed? The U.S.S.R. counter-claims to provide means of production, distribution and sale within the control of all its people, who never the less do not enjoy that half of the fruits of their labour dissipated on armaments. A degree of inscrutability which would exceed caricature has until recently obscured the fate of the Chinese, but with that admittedly massive exception, most countries in the world could be classified somewhere between doctrinaire communism and laissez-faire capitalism.

Throughout the world, however, an increasing search for personal satisfaction disrupts the otherwise placid atmosphere engendered by the *status quo*! The generation gap appears, or perhaps is only more loudly recognised. Younger people protest about the system, and blame their elders for its existence. The "establishment", even though it may itself have been revolutionary, attracts criticism and violence, and adopts or increases violent repression. Without expressing any political judgement, it is possible to recognise the anguish of the protesting Czech communist waving his Party card, and the bewilderment of the Russian soldier he confronts, who believes himself to be "supporting" the Czech people. Closer to home the chronic unemployment and resulting deprivation of opportunity for a constructive pasttime is recognised as one of the several factors predisposing to the violence now current in Northern Ireland.

Students question the nature of society, while being supported by provisions made for them by that society. While the ranks of ageing protestors is swelled by recruits both young and old, pressures to change numerous aspects of society build up, but this increasing tempo of destruction is not accompanied by any crescendo of constructive alternative proposals. Are humans the victims of forces they are unable to control?

A group who discussed this question first considered the part that industry might play. In their role as members of commercial enterprises, they soon saw that industry as such would not materially affect society for the better (but see below), perhaps because it produced what that consuming society demands, either in terms of comestibles or satisfactory stock market performance. Thus projecting the problem on to political associations, they felt able to indicate objectively individual needs, and the means by which society might satisfy them. In this context, "society" is not synonymous with "the State", though at times, society worked through State agencies.

Taking Maslow's hierarchy of needs as a framework, it was seen that Society, not "them", or Parliament, or the Church, but *we* have to work towards providing food and shelter for everyone. At the time of writing a national dock strike has led to a shortage of essential supplies in the Scottish Isles. Dockers who volunteer to load ships are entitled to some pay for their labour, for "why should they do their usual work for nothing." At the same time, these dockers do not want to be at an advantage over their fellows drawing only strike pay, so they pass the wage they earn to charity. Because they have been paid, state security benefits to which the dockers' families are entitled (for it is not the wives and children who are in the dispute) are stopped, and an injustice is suffered by those not directly concerned. Negotiation results in a compromise by which the wages earned are paid directly to the nominated charity. The dockers receive nothing, and the legal niceties of social security benefits are complied with. Note that the important associated factor here is the society which makes such a compromise possible and acceptable.

Increasing attention is being paid to the preservation of life, and its quality. Some of the countries that lead the world in production capability now consider whether they are saturated with cars, or consumer products. The principle of "built-in obsolescence" to maintain production is questioned, and there are moves both to husband limited raw materials, and to dispose of waste in a way which does not detract from the quality of life. Society, like the soul, begins to exhibit a conscience.

Perhaps a more contentious activity is the attempt to limit population. Motives for doing so can be obscure to the eye of the beholder, whose underdeveloped country is the main target for propaganda. The "have nots" have hitherto provided for the exigencies of their precarious existence by procreating sufficient children to survive the risks of primitive life. Is it not perverse that an early benefit bestowed upon them with some generosity, is the medical skill that makes matters worse, by helping too many to survive?

To back up the conscience of society, legislation is expected to elicit conformity with rules, and to inculcate into the individual some desirable attributes. Safety legislation blossomed in Britain in the wake of the industrial revolution and its associated dangers. At first the weak found refuge from the strong, and the employed were protected from their employer. Now limitations upon alcohol consumption when driving protects us from each other, and in some countries, car seat belt legislation protects us from ourselves.

Security needs are catered for by a society which increasingly abhors, or fears, outright war. Countries now attempt to reconcile conflicting national aims, to preserve those aspects of society common to them all, such as a standard of living. The Common Market starts as an economic arrangement, but leads to mutual recognition of aspirations of the peoples concerned. Currency control protects the economy, but also prevents a slump and repetition of the misery and frustrations of the returned heroes who were unemployed in the thirties. Consumer interests are protected by legislation against unfair practices in hire purchase, money lending and mortgages. Insurance is in some instances compulsory, whether in the public or private sector, so that an accident's effect upon an individual or his family is not devastating.

Less easy to deal with are the love and belonging needs. Victorians depended upon "a circle of friends" for their informal leisure activity, and though radio, cinema, and television widen perspective enormously, they can isolate as well. Provision of radio for the blind, or television for the disabled, doubtless counters their isolation, but television can smother interaction between those watching it. Paradoxically, the family that stays at home and watches television as if it were "moving wallpaper" may communicate less with each other than before. Children may gain education through that medium, but they may lack contact with parents whose "telly" they may not disturb! Moreover, as society becomes more materialistic, broken homes (or even some intact ones) tend to demonstrate less love and caring for children who are overwhelmed with material gifts, toys, or money, instead of enjoying the real interest of their parents.

A striking feature of immigrant populations is the contrast they demonstrate between their extended, and the host countries' nuclear-families. Migration from agriculture to the towns breaks up long established groupings, and life in the city may provide only two sets of relationships—the immediate family, and the work group. Loss of a job may isolate the whole family, as well as depriving it of sustenance. Immigrants from further afield have difficulties of language and culture, isolation, membership of a minority group, perhaps in terms of religion as well as race.[31] They tend to become scapegoats, in that they may be pressured into menial tasks, with low pay whatever their capability. They are therefore more dependent upon their work than the host community, put up with worse conditions, and are then blamed for not supporting action to improve those conditions.

When one considers the host society's nuclear family, one recognises the implied number of lonely people. Where before, grandparents cared for small children while young adults supported both, today's pattern is for the State to provide nurseries and old people's homes, so that the productive workers can both work, and enjoy their leisure. How often does the general practitioner in Britain hear the phrase "Dad (or Mum) is getting on a bit now, will you please arrange for him to go into hospital?" Society shares the individual's responsibility for this lack of affection, because council homes have been designed for half a century as if there were never to be a need to house an elderly relative. Fortunately, efforts are now being made to preserve the independence and dignity of the aged, while yet caring for their needs, by provision of accommodation where there is a warden to look out for illness or difficulty. One local authority goes even further in providing accommodation not only for the workers it hopes to attract, but for some of the elderly dependants who might otherwise be left behind.

Ego needs have only recently enjoyed any attempt at satisfaction, and the most notable examples have been initiated by the workers themselves rather than by anyone else. In Scotland, workers on the Clyde successfully forced society to recognise not only their need for work, but the skills and reputations of which they were proud. By refusing to be dispersed, and by coming to terms with the new situation, helped by Government subsidy, the shipbuilders have gained respite from the march of events which might otherwise have priced them out of the market. It will be interesting to see whether the admiration of society will be justified by subsequently continued productive "status" drives. Certainly, admiration from one quarter demands justification from the other.

Self-actualisation needs might be better served by greater effort to recognise the enormous untapped reserve of individual ability. While appreciation by one's superiors might satisfy the ego, the opportunity to exercise one's skill is essential. Both managers and the managed should receive education and training to appreciate not only the ecological environment, but to recognise a toxic psychological environment. This might well lead to a reversal of some deeply instilled British traditions. At school the perfidy of sneaking is clear, but the person who copes with stress by heavy drinking of alcohol may depend upon someone "sneaking" about him for his survival, dependent of course upon an atmosphere in which constructive help rather than immediate dismissal will ensue. Those interested in the problems must take every opportunity to use all means of communication. Not only companies, but whole populations and governments should have their attention drawn to these problems. Pressure groups concerned with aircraft noise are but one example.

It is interesting to note that the Windsor seminar group which debated the subject of this chapter, considered that new towns should pay more attention to the social needs of the isolated or elderly. They saw a role which might be played by social clubs sponsored by firms moving into or already established in development areas. Moreover, the opportunities offered to design new factories to allow for greater self-actualisation were identified by the group, which may not have realised that they had thus contradicted their starting point—namely the assumption that industry can do little to alleviate the ills of society (see page 137).

Since the Windsor seminar took place, some of the changes which could be foreseen have taken place, and some of the remedies there suggested have been put into practice by others who had apparently reached similar conclusions independently.

As the European Economic Community enlarges, it will be interesting to see to what extent the threat of change, and the defensive consolidation of practice already locally established, will counteract the increasing capability of some individuals for change. If political manoeuvring can be separated from manipulation of circumstances to provide the satisfactions the whole Economic Community will require, the wider range of opportunity, the increase in the standard of living, and the structure of the society which develops, may hasten the achievement of some of the objectives of the young protestors of today. There will almost certainly be further approximation of the capitalist and socialist systems which has already begun, because trade, communication and cultural exchanges must lead towards equilibrium within, rather than balance between, the main blocs now divided by a rusting curtain.

Lest that remark be dismissed as an idle, naive hope, it is worth directing attention to one example of a problem common to all industrial societies. Elsewhere, the need to re-examine our society's assumptions and self-deceptions concerning absenteeism has been demonstrated. Yugoslavia has similar experience, despite the contrasting ideology.

In that country, one occupational physician was asked to investigate a sudden rise in absenteeism over a three month period in one department of a furniture factory, managed by a workers' council. At first, some feature of the furniture polishing process was suspected as being the cause, but when records were examined, only two out of seventy people were found to be suffering from demonstrable organic disease. Apart from a few colds, all other absences, characteristically lasting for between one to three days, were found to be ascribed to headaches, lumbago, painful periods, stomach upsets, and dizziness; that is to say they were psychosomatic explanations for absence.

Careful study of the process indicated that there had been no change in materials or methods, but a new foreman had been in office for the period in question. He had been elected by his fellows because he had always been critical of supervisors. He had been very popular as a workmate, and had both skill and long experience. Once elected, he had changed entirely, to become authoritative, and to be despised by his erstwhile colleagues. Some of them came into conflict with him, others avoided his attention and others avoided him completely by "flight into sickness". A disagreeable instance of his management style led the workers' council to enquire into the behaviour and opinions of other foremen, and it was decided that the foremen should meet together to discuss their problems.

A framework for discussion was established by a brief account of various management styles and illustrations of interpersonal relations. Nonetheless it was necessary to allow the foremen to absorb this information by discussion and explanation of their own experiences. At an early stage, antipathy between older and younger men became apparent. Older men had experienced authoritarian management in the past, which had helped to determine their own style. "Where would we end if youngsters were allowed to have their way?" was a typical remark, which necessitated explanation of the difference between freedom and licence, and of the limitations of democracy.

This led to expression of doubts as to the relevance of such a group discussion. The older men present feared criticism by the younger, who in their turn became silent, perhaps in order to run less risk of being accused of impertinence, or of provoking trouble. So the whole group was asked to list the risks that would arise if a group of workers were allowed to make their own decision through group discussions. "Impudent, long haired youths", or "workers not fit to work with", or the especially difficult lorry drivers were mentioned, and conversation progressed to include *assumptions* people make about each other. In this case, worker and foremen had fears of each other's intentions. The foremen's concern was that if people were allowed to decide for themselves, they would take advantage of the situation to diminish discipline and to avoid working if possible. Organisation would become confused, responsibility would be shelved and production would fall off. When all these fears had been spoken, the foremen became less aggressive, and it is important to note that this lessening of tension could not have been imposed. Relaxation could only be derived *from within the group itself.*

Now "unfrozen" members of the group, whether young or old, could reach some conclusions. They could now appreciate what everyone knows, namely that if efficiency and income depended upon their own discipline, workers would be serious and industrious. Work and responsibility distributed in relation to each task by the self-disciplined group would become less onerous. (Family businesses all over the world have demonstrated this for centuries. It is also worth noting that some skilled shift workers in Britain have less absenteeism than day workers, perhaps because they answer to each other for the increased work load of those who do turn up!) From that self-discipline, organisation of tasks and responsibilities would emerge, and if the foreman were a team leader, he would support and be supported by his group in the exercise of responsibility. Since all would contribute to the discipline, and participate in the allocation of jobs, productivity and quality would be likely to increase, so leading to a higher income. One foreman summed up, "Let them work hard to see how hard it is for us!"

This account has been included to illustrate that human drives and instincts transcend ideological barriers constructed by differing societies, each of which may well have assumed that "they don't have that problem" or that "we don't have that problem". Foremen in Britain have been described as "the meat in the sandwich", and foremen and forewomen are not necessarily comparable even within the same company, because of the prejudices of society as a whole. The need to dispel prejudice is equalled by the need for education and understanding. The role of managers has to be learnt, and divorced from the class distinction of our society.

17

Whose Responsibility?

WHILE semantic definition of stress is difficult recognition of the state of internal stress can be intuitively accurate within the limits set out earlier in this book.

Society, as the conscience of a community, has to overcome the prejudice it displays towards mental strain and illness. A man may break his leg and be away from work for months, while his employer and colleagues await the inexorable progress of organic repair, eventually to welcome him back to his former post. How different is the reaction to breakdown of mental composure. A period off work, during which readjustment restores mental equilibrium, may be less than the time necessary for repair of a fracture of both bones of the lower leg; yet the limp evokes sympathy, while restored mental balance is viewed with reserve, permanent weakness is suspected, and the disability which may be a fantasy of the beholder becomes a permanent stigma to be borne by him who suffered only transient mental injury.

Industrialised communities have become more enlightened in recent years, and commercial organisations attempt to promote or preserve mental wellbeing in a number of ways, which vary greatly, but may be described as being distributed along a continuum between two extremes. At one end of the spectrum, increasing complexity of the organisation and its problems suggests the multiplication of specialists in narrow fields. At the other extreme a "jack of all trades" approach is preferred, so that training is widely dispersed, across a wider field of subjects, but with a lesser degree of competence.

The former approach was preferred by a Dutch businessman at the Windsor seminar, and seemed to reflect industrial practice in larger firms in Holland.

The hypothesis was that the successful commercial structure was supported by two main pillars, which represented continuity and production. Each pillar was itself made up of several columns, so that "production" consisted of all those departments directed towards that end, such as technical, sales, marketing and distribution. The continuity of the enterprise depended upon the recruitment of labour, the calculation of wages, the legal obligations of the company itself, and these functions were carried out by specialists in law, or in personnel management. To existing specialism it was suggested that another be added, to be called the Social Department, with the objective of making sure that proper relationships should exist between those within a department, or between different departments, as a task in itself. It was recognised that this function might already be performed by more traditional personnel departments in some, but not all, firms. One large British firm has a comparable structure, which to some extent answers the rhetorical question "Who guards those who are on guard?", but an important feature of the Dutch model was the executive power enjoyed by specialists whose powers would be restricted in Britain to the proffering of advice.

There seems to be a paradox in the tendency to multiply the specialists who care for various functions of people, when the tendency to reduce those people's jobs into separate simple parts is now being reversed to allow sufficient exercise of skill to satisfy the person. The "jack of all trades" approach seemed to commend itself more to the British managers, who felt that rather than to delegate responsibilities to specialists, everyone who had charge of others should have training in, and responsibility for the welfare and working conditions of his subordinates. Just as a greater level of education was reversing the trend towards ever simpler repetitive tasks, so should the manager be expected to have a higher level of understanding.

There is a similarity between that challenge and the one facing the medical profession in Britain. About 600 doctors have a specific responsibility for the occupational health of the 26,000,000 people who go out to work. Not only is there a need for interest among those doctors to be widened beyond traditional physical and chemical toxicology; the 50,000 doctors in general practice and hospitals need to acquire a greater understanding of the community as a whole, and of the work their patients do.

While this wider interest has to be promoted in the medical profession, managers and the community at large have to be helped to perceive that health is a matter closely related to very many aspects of commerce and life in general. With roots spread over so wide an area, the relevance of some of the traditional compartments of interest need review.

In industry, the occupational physician's role may require him to be a medically qualified manager, who applies to the problem of business views derived from his medical knowledge. The proposal is controversial, since such a doctor may appear to abandon traditional detachment from mercenary pursuits. Even in his present role, his motives are suspect, and perhaps the suspicion can only be dispelled by greater contact between him and his colleagues, on both a social and a professional level. Some attempts are already made to achieve this, by providing facilities for the investigation of patients on behalf of their own doctors. In this way co-operative concern for the patient is expressed.

The danger of assuming that a specialist necessarily has managerial competence has already been noted. The individualist practitioner has been formally recognised in the British Social Security system by conferring upon each principal general practitioner the status of independent contractor. This objective was to maintain independent clinical freedom as a duly qualified medical practitioner, but the degree of independence has been exaggerated to the point at which he answers to no one for his performance, unless he kills or seduces a patient! His whole training has been to equip him to take sole responsibility for his actions.

A further burden of his training is his conditioning to react to pathology or to cries for help, and his rules of etiquette deter him from offering spontaneous advice. When approached, he is treated by the patient with deference, and is expected to give pontifical advice; he can easily fall into an attitude of mind in which he feels more at home giving "divine" orders than in consciously expressing a fallible opinion. There are some who suggest that a process of self-selection leads certain doctors to practice in industry because they prefer to work in an environment which they cannot find in other branches of medicine.

If the doctor has a conflict of roles, so do those he works among have conflicts in their attitudes to him. The problem of being perceived as an agent of the employer while practising in a traditionally ethical manner has been discussed. An even greater problem is posed by any claim he may make to management skills, because he may then threaten others who preferred him to stick to *their* concept of medicine. When once a doctor advised an engineer upon the technical specifications and installation of a machine which might be a noise hazard, the engineer expressed the view that the doctor should confine his attention to ears, for the machine was the engineer's business! How much more difficult it is for the manager to be advised by a doctor on how to organise his department, or how to handle a particular subordinate or even a whole department.

Yet this is the scale of the challenge of the maintenance of mental health in industry. Specialists, whether in personnel, technical or medical departments, have to become accustomed to working as members of a team. Each has to earn the right to give advice to his colleagues by establishing and demonstrating his own competence, and contribute to the training of their successors; and that implies that the doctor has a role to play in management training. At the simplest level, it is already ridiculous that any manager or foreman should call for a first aider to treat one of those in his care, and yet it is common experience that the foreman or manager receives no training whatever for coping with any accident or emergency. Indeed both managements and unions look to medical departments to provide emergency care, blissfully unaware that for the real emergency, three minutes is the maximum time limit upon the response. What is the sense of having a nurse on duty twenty-four hours a day, if she is employed only to establish legal provision of an "adequate" number of first aid boxes and first aid trained personnel? Those legal per capita provisions are already notoriously out of date even in terms of the equipment demanded, and reflect an attitude to first aid that is as out of date as Florence Nightingale herself would be.

Should he express such a view, the occupational physician could become involved in fundamental reappraisal of the medical department's role by both management and unions, and is likely to be accused of abdicating his responsibilities, while claiming others. The trades union official may well see himself as the only apostle of progress and social justice, and may indeed presently fulfil some of the needs of those about him for counselling and advice.

Earlier chapters have mentioned the suspicion doctors and psychologists attracted by becoming involved in the Swedish mental health campaign. When they heard of the proposal to computerise a very wide range of personnel information in the Philips company, doctors had expressed considerable reservations about the ethical standards of computer staff, and those who had access to the computer. Both reactions may have been concern that individual integrity or status might be undermined, and this reaction may well have been experienced by the reader at various places in this book, where he finds himself expected to undertake more in some fields and less in others.

Both management and union training schemes should now direct attention to the control of stress

1. by educating and training people to cope with challenge
2. by better control of a crisis when it occurs
3. by intervention in the sequel to crisis
4. by assisting the individual to recover after breakdown has occurred.

The Trades Union Congress already includes some of these topics in courses run at Congress House for shop stewards. The Industrial Society and British Institute of Management have also organised seminars and conferences, but in the latter cases it is remarkable that the invitation to participate always settles finally on the desk of someone in the personnel or medical departments. Thus, for management, direction of attention to stress is preached to the converted. Until people become aware they have a problem, they do not seek help, and the purpose of this chapter has been to help the reader to awareness. Answers to his problem are likely to be valid only if he himself contributes to its identification and solution.

Conclusion

IN Britain, approximately 7,000,000 people work in factories, and less than 2,000,000 of those work in the 800 or so factories employing more than 1,000 staff. Unions have an approximate membership of 10,000,000 and many of these are drawn from the total working population, not just those working in factories. These figures imply much about the total environment of the adult population.

Six hundred full-time occupational physicians care for the larger working groups represented by those 2,000,000 workers in factories large enough to have justified provision of medical care at work. Approximately 2,000 out of the 24,000 general practitioners in Britain practice any form of industrial medicine. Only a handful of academic or hospital doctors have ever been in a factory.

The vast majority of members of the medical and ancillary professions need education and training in the understanding of health at work, and until it is made available to them, 24,000,000 people spend one-third of their lives in activities which attract little or no formal medical interest.

It has been said that "if a whole man is employed, his managers and doctors are inevitably concerned with his total environment". However, the Robens Report[32] concludes that there is little justification for a comprehensive occupational health service since there would be duplication of services already the responsibility of the National Health Service—but the Report's paragraphs on Occupational Health Services state there is no recognition of anything other than organic disease. A gleam of hope may be visible in the recognition by the Royal College of General Practitioners that training of future general practitioners should include consideration of the total psycho-social environment.

A vast population works in units "too small to justify a personnel department". While it is true that the larger organisations have greater problems of communication and understanding which obviously require personnel expertise, there must be an enormous number of people working in groups too big to enjoy the familiarity and close knit conditions in which problems are solved intuitively, while yet being too small to contain even one manager who has the time or duty to study human relationships. These workers and managers may not even be aware that they have group or individual problems. In some ways that may appear to be a blessing, but in the longer term, the interplay between those small groups and the larger groups with which they are in competition for work, housing, or leisure facilities is likely to lead to individual or group breakdown.

An apathetic and vast majority needs education in human relationships, so that prejudices of class, creed or race can be explained, understood, and resolved. The attempt to provide such understanding in Sweden was perceived by some employers as being dangerous and some of the employed (and perhaps the reader) will suspect that aspiration as being a call to revolution, rather than as a recognition of a process of evolution.

The Army, the Law, and the Church are no longer pre-eminent among the professions. The distinction between a "professional" man and a "business" man is much less. Perhaps evolution in the best tradition of British life will lead towards a situation brought about in China with scant regard or compassion for individuals of the old order.

In a recent paper,[33] a European doctor working in China described how care for the rural population is shared by its members. No one was exempted by considerations of status from the need to do manual work for a time each year. Moreover, even those men who would be "professional" in Europe are expected to be participants in the general life of the local community, rather than to be accorded the privilege of exclusive exercise of their specialism. The paper dealt in particular with medical care in a developing country, and described how one person in a village would be sent off from time to time to study first aid, primary medical care, elementary public health and similar topics. Some of these people would remain at a very low level of competence indefinitely, but those who were capable of doing so continued to receive intermittent training and constant practical experience and appraisal until they became qualified as doctors in either Western or traditional Chinese medicine, both of which exist side by side.

While the method of achieving this state of affairs is open to question, the feasibility of greater participation in the total life of the community, without loss of technical competence is demonstrated. It may be that some of the conflicts familiar to us might be resolved by reducing the number and rigidity of the compartments into which industrialised societies are divided.

Various disciplines, and within particular disciplines, opposing schools of thought have put forward ideas about stress. Most doctors recognise stress disease, but disagree about the conditions which might be grouped under that heading. Psychologists postulate hypotheses, which can be opposed as cogently as they are proposed. Behavioural scientists vary in the marketing ability they display in presenting their syllabuses for training managers. Hewers of wood and drawers of water tend to dismiss the lot as airy-fairy nonsense without relevance to them.

It is surely remarkable that measures thought appropriate at Hawthorne, or management philosophies propounded by Glacier Metals Ltd., or the Managerial Grid, or other "solutions" to the personnel problems in industry do not gain widespread support. Can it be because organisations differ so much that experience cannot be extrapolated from one place to another? Perhaps some basic assumptions are not questioned sufficiently. Certainly few attempts have been made to identify the positive qualities of small enterprises to identify those characteristics which might be energetically preserved as the enterprise itself grows in complexity. Perhaps there is an analogy here between the doctors training to respond to pathology, rather than to investigate what it is that keeps his patient healthy.

There are many more post mortems on companies that have failed, than there are explanations for those that succeed. There are virtually no therapeutic trials to quantify "before" and "after" situations, to assess the result in terms of people, of a change in commercial activity. There is a need for research into some of the basic assumptions about stress. What evidence is there that environmental factors are more important than personal defects in the incidence of breakdown?

Attention has repeatedly been drawn to the gap between those who manage and those managed. It is a bizarre twist of fate that those who are convinced that all humans should have equal dignity and opportunity, find themselves addressing almost exclusively those who have taken opportunity and established their dignity. That statement in no sense questions the sincerity of the various apostles. Their training language, and even sometimes the jargon they compose, make them incomprehensible to those very people who deserve their greatest interest. Moreover, frequent reference to "management" problems is perceived only in the "superior" sense, and is not appreciated in its significance by the "subordinates", who form the other half of the picture. There is a need for "translation" of much of behavioural science into plain language.

The concept of sectional interest extends beyond management and the managed into the community as a whole. The demarcation dispute between doctors and "the rest", in which doctors claim, or are assumed to have, exclusive responsibility or competence in matters of mental health has received attention elsewhere, but deserves repetition. After all, the second generation of man posed the question "Am I my brother's keeper?" and the answer was apparently long before John Donne composed that fine response—"No man is an island . . ."

Appendix I

References

(including Further Reading List)

1. Maslow, A. H., *Motivation and Personality* (Harper, New York, 1954)
2. Herzberg, F., Mausner, B., Snyderman, B., *The Motivation to Work*, (John Wiley, New York; Chapman & Hall, London, 1966)
3. *Management Today*, January '73, British Institute of Management, London
4. Laurence, J., Hull, R., *The Peter Principle* (Souvenir Press, London, 1969)
5. Emery, F. E. and Trist, E. L., *The Causal Texture of Organisational Environment* (Human Relations, 1965, *18* Vol. I)
6. Hudson, L., *Intelligence, divergence, and potential originality*, (Nature 1962, *196*, No. 4854, 601–602)
7. Fraser, R., *Work*, 2 volumes (an edited series of essays by workers) a Pelican book (Penguin Books, Harmondsworth, Middlesex)
8. Flanders, A., *The Fawley Productivity Agreements* (Faber & Faber Ltd., London, 1964)
9. Sergean, R., *Managing Shiftwork* (Gower Press Limited, 1971)
10. Bion, W. R., *Experiences in Groups* (Tavistock, 1961)
11. Dalton, Katherina, *The Menstrual Cycle* (Penguin, 1969)
12. Dominian, J., *Marital Breakdown* (Pelican, 1969)
13. Gillon, J. J., *Toronto ou la rencontre* (Le Concours Medical, September, 1954)
14. McGregor, D., *The Human Side of Enterprise* (McGraw-Hill, 1960)

15. Symposium (1968) *Absence from work attributed to sickness*, (Proceedings published by Research Panel, Society of Occupational Medicine, London)
16. Herzberg, F., Mausner, B., Petersen, R., Capwell, D., *Job Attitudes: review of research and opinions* (Pittsburg, 1967)
17. Hill, J. M. M., Trist, E. L., (1955) *Changes in accidents and other absences with length of service* (Human Relations 8 Tavistock pamphlet No. 4)
18. Hinkle, L. E., Wolff, H. G., (1957) *The nature of man's adaptation to his total environment, and the relation of this to illness* (Arch. Intern. Med. *99*, 442–460)
19. Ekker, W. (1965) *Some experience with diagnosis statistics in a group of Dutch industries* (2nd International Conference on sick absence statistics, Amsterdam)
20. de Groot, M. J. W. (1965) 2nd International Conference on Sick Absence Statistics, Amsterdam
21. Chiesman, W. E., (1957) *Clinical aspects of Absenteeism* (Royal Society of Health Journal, *77*, 681–689)
22. Buzzard, R. B., Shaw, W. J. (1952) *Analysis of absence under a scheme of paid sick leave* (B.J.I.M. *9*, 282–295)
23. Ennals, Rt. Hon. David (1969) Dept. of Health and Social Security, London
24. Ashworth, H. W. (1957) M.D. Thesis, University of Manchester
25. Samuel, P. J., (1969) *Labour turnover—towards a solution* Institute of Personel Management
26. Raffle, A. (1970) *The Occupational Physician as the Community Physician* (Presidential Address, Occupational Medicine Section, Royal Society of Medicine, London)
27. Philips Industries, *Work Structuring* (an illustrated booklet in English available on request from Dr. J. Doeglas)
28. Mindus, E., *Work and Mental Health* (available in Swedish, but English translation in preparation)
29. Amark, C., *The Individual, Personality and Human Environment* (available only in Swedish)
30. Blake, R., Moulton, J. S., *The Managerial Grid* (Gulf Publishing Co., Houston, Texas, 1964)

31. Verhaegen, P., *Mental Health in Foreign Workers*, Acco, 1972, Leuven, Belgium

32. The Robens Report *Health and Safety at Work* (H.M.S.O., 1972)

33. Ciba Foundation Blueprint *Teamwork for World Health* (J. & A. Churchill, 1971)

Appendix II

A Glossary of Terms

Definitions taken from English H.B. and English A.G., *A Comprehensive Dictionary of Psychological and Psycho-Analytical Terms*:

COGNITION   any process whereby an organism becomes aware or obtains knowledge of an object. In most systems, cognition, affection and conation are the three categories under which all mental processes are classified. Adjective—cognitive; verb—cognise.

CONTENT ANALYSIS   discovering and listing according to a systematic plan the ideas, feelings, truth claims and personal references in a communication.

EXPERIENTIAL   the process or experience of actual living through an event or events.

PROCESS   a change or a changing in an object or organism in which a consistent quality or direction can be discerned. Both physiology and psychology are primarily sciences of process.

PROJECTION   the process of unwittingly attributing one's own traits, attitudes or subjective processes to others.

Index